HEALTH CARE ISSUES, COSTS AND ACCESS

QUALITY IMPROVEMENT

METHODS, PRINCIPLES AND ROLE IN HEALTHCARE

HEALTH CARE ISSUES, COSTS AND ACCESS

Additional books in this series can be found on Nova's website under the Series tab.

Additional E-books in this series can be found on Nova's website under the E-book tab.

HEALTH CARE ISSUES, COSTS AND ACCESS

QUALITY IMPROVEMENT

METHODS, PRINCIPLES AND ROLE IN HEALTHCARE

KEVIN W. LOBDELL
AND
SOTIRIS C. STAMOU
EDITORS

nova publishers
New York

Library of Congress Cataloging-in-Publication Data

Library of Congress Control Number: 2012952788

ISBN: 978-1-62417-390-5

Published by Nova Science Publishers, Inc. † New York

Contents

SECTION ONE: NATIONAL INITIATIVES

In: Quality Improvement
Editors: K. W. Lobdell and S. C. Stamou
ISBN: 978-1-62417-390-5

Chapter 1

HEALTHCARE QUALITY IMPROVEMENT FROM A NATIONAL AND REGIONAL LEVEL

Mark Stewart and Sara Camp*

American Heart Association/American Stroke Association – National Center, Dallas, TX, US

ABSTRACT

Founded in 1924, with our more than 20 million supporters and volunteers, both professional and lay, the American Heart Association/American Stroke Association (AHA/ASA) is a trusted and credible source for science and for quality improvement (QI). The Mission of the AHA/ASA is *Building healthier lives free of cardiovascular disease and stroke.* The AHA/ASA's 2020 impact goal is to improve the cardiovascular health of all Americans by 20% while reducing deaths from CVD and stroke by 20% by 2020. In order to reach the aforementioned goals, the AHA/ASA dedicates considerable efforts towards healthcare QI. Proudly, the AHA has served as an innovator in quality and in particular, in QI programs, for over 10 years. The flagship of our efforts is centered on the Get With The Guidelines® (Get With The Guidelines) in-hospital QI program, a program which now has over 1900 hospitals nationwide leveraging its tools and resources. With those 1900 hospitals has also come a wealth of data and patient records. Currently, over 3.6 million patients have been touched by the efforts of these hospitals to improve care for their patients.

One of AHA/ASA's approaches to its mission is to continually raise the bar on quality patient care by advocating for and creating systems, programs, and partnerships that ensure that evidence-based medical guidelines are effectively translated into standard patient care. AHA/ASA has developed the premier answer to innovative healthcare change and can drive massive penetration of programs proven to improve quality of patient care, improve short-term outcomes and eliminate healthcare disparities. The AHA/ASA has served as a pioneer in healthcare quality and QI programs, marked by published, peer-reviewed evidence of success, for more than two decades, setting us apart from other patient and professional organizations. As previously mentioned, the flagship of these efforts has been the Get With The Guidelines suite of in-hospital QI programs which have impacted the care of more than 3 million patients and resulted in over 4 million patient records. Get With The Guidelines is the largest national hospital-based

* E-mail: sara.camp@heart.org.

program dedicated to quality of care improvement for patients with cardiovascular disease. The objectives of the Get With The Guidelines program are to:

- Improve care and education of patients hospitalized with CVD and Stroke
- Accelerate initiation of the evidence-based, guideline-recommended therapies in appropriate patients without contraindications
- Enhance management of comorbidities and related risks
- Facilitate coordination of care, transitions of care and outpatient follow-up

INTRODUCTION

Founded in 1924, with our more than 20 million supporters and volunteers, both professional and lay, the American Heart Association/ American Stroke Association (AHA/ASA) is a trusted and credible source for science and for quality improvement (QI). The Mission of the AHA/ASA is *Building healthier lives free of cardiovascular disease and stroke.* The AHA/ASA's 2020 impact goal is to improve the cardiovascular health of all Americans by 20% while reducing deaths from CVD and stroke by 20% by 2020. In order to reach the aforementioned goals, the AHA/ASA dedicates considerable efforts towards healthcare QI. Proudly, the AHA has served as an innovator in quality and in particular, in QI programs, for over 10 years. The flagship of our efforts is centered on the Get With The Guidelines® (Get With The Guidelines) in-hospital QI program, a program which now has over 1900 hospitals nationwide leveraging its tools and resources. With those 1900 hospitals has also come a wealth of data and patient records. Currently, over 3.6 million patients have been touched by the efforts of these hospitals to improve care for their patients.

Currently, the AHA/ASA is comprised of seven regional affiliates spanning the United States with the National Center in Dallas, Texas and a federal advocacy office in Washington, DC. The AHA is committed to increased research, improved access to quality treatment and targeted and reinvigorated efforts directed at primordial and primary prevention. Science application is accelerated by offering health information and solutions to consumers, professionals and media; advocating for public policy and systems change to promote healthier environments, improve earlier diagnosis and management of cardiovascular health factors, and enhance systems of care to better prevent and treat CVD and stroke; and working to reduce and eliminate disparities in managing health and improving quality care.

AHA's Executive Leadership Committee is comprised of chief executive officer, chief mission officer, chief administrative officer, chief development officer, chief science officer, and affiliate executive vice presidents which all have performance standards related to Get With The Guidelines, tied to the number of hospitals achieving award recognition levels.

PROGRAMS (OVERVIEW)

One of AHA/ASA's approaches to its mission is to continually raise the bar on quality patient care by advocating for and creating systems, programs, and partnerships that ensure that evidence-based medical guidelines are effectively translated into standard patient care.

Table 1. Quality Improvement Programs

	Year Initiated	Number of Hospitals, Systems or Physician Practices Participating	Total Patients Entered	Total Patient Records Entered
Get With The Guidelines-CAD	2000	n/a	563,407	615,184
ACTION Registry-GWTG	2008	706	n/a	358,379
Get With The Guidelines-Heart Failure	2005	550	581,901	696,382
Get With The Guidelines-Stroke	2003	1640	2,069,448	2,140,434
Get With The Guidelines-Resuscitation	2000	296	415,029	493,062
Totals		3,192	3,629,785	4,303,441
The Guideline Advantage Physician Practices	2009	9	167,590	1,147,015
Target: Stroke Registered	2010	1,373	n/a	n/a
Target: Heart Failure Registered	2011	238	n/a	n/a
Mission: Lifeline STEMI Systems Registered	2007	606	n/a	n/a
Hospital Accreditation and Certification Mission: Lifeline STEMI Receiving Centers	2011	11	n/a	n/a
The Joint Commission – Primary Stroke Center (AHA/ASA)	2003	943	n/a	n/a
The Joint Commission AHA Advanced Certification in Heart Failure	2009	41	n/a	n/a
Totals			3,797,375	5,450,456

AHA/ASA has developed the premier answer to innovative healthcare change and can drive massive penetration of programs proven to improve quality of patient care, improve short-term outcomes and eliminate healthcare disparities.

The AHA/ASA has served as a pioneer in healthcare quality and QI programs, marked by published, peer-reviewed evidence of success, for more than two decades, setting us apart from other patient and professional organizations. As previously mentioned, the flagship of these efforts has been the Get With The Guidelines suite of in-hospital QI programs which have impacted the care of more than 3 million patients and resulted in over 4 million patient records. Get With The Guidelines is the largest national hospital-based program dedicated to quality of care improvement for patients with cardiovascular disease. The objectives of the Get With The Guidelines program are to:

- Improve care and education of patients hospitalized with CVD and Stroke
- Accelerate initiation of the evidence-based, guideline-recommended therapies in appropriate patients without contraindications
- Enhance management of comorbidities and related risks
- Facilitate coordination of care, transitions of care and outpatient follow-up

Focus on Quality

Quality Improvement Programs Weekly Overview Summary - October 8, 2012				
	Year Initiated	Number of Hospitals, Systems or Physicians' Practices Participating	Total Patients Entered	Total Patient Records Entered
GWTG-CAD*	2000	n/a	563,407	615,184
ACTION-Registry-GWTG	2008	779	n/a	358,379
GWTG-HF	2005	559	613,878	737,802
GWTG-Stroke	2003	1,642	2,184,043	2,277,007
GWTG-Resuscitation	2000	298	437,310	520,399
Totals		3,278	3,798,638	4,508,771
The Guideline Advantage Physician Practices	2009	33	246,350	1,521,669
Target: Stroke Registered	2010	1,484	n/a	n/a
Target: Heart Failure Registered	2011	301	n/a	n/a
Mission: Lifeline STEMI Systems Registered	2007	648	n/a	n/a
Hospital Accreditation & Certification				
Mission: Lifeline STEMI Receiving Centers	2011	14	n/a	n/a
The Joint Commission - Primary Stroke Center (AHA/ASA)	2003	994	n/a	n/a
The Joint Commission AHA Advanced Certification in Heart Failure	2009	41	n/a	n/a
Totals			4,044,988	6,030,440

GWTG-CAD: Program completed transition to ACTION-Registry GWTG 12/31/09*

Figure 1. American Heart Association/American Stroke Focus on Quality Suite of Programs Nationwide Peneration.

There are many other registry programs in the country, but one important distinction of the AHA's Get With The Guidelines is the aspect of continuous QI. Two key aspects of CQI are eliminating unnecessary variation and spreading innovations. Through the research conducted on data from Get With The Guidelines and the 175+ peer-reviewed manuscripts generated from the data, variations in care can be identified and innovations can be spread. It is more than mere collection and reporting of results by providing benchmark reports and suggestions for small tests of change. Rather than just a "Plan-Do-Study-Publish" model, the Get With The Guidelines represent a true "Plan-Do-Study-Act" approach.

At the community level, hospitals receive consultation from QI (QI) directors to help identify opportunities for improvement and facilitate inter-hospital sharing of best practices. QI directors continually analyze hospital performance data to determine what performance metrics need attention at any given time. Because many participating hospitals do not come to the program with QI experience, the quality programs cultivate these skills and culture in participating sites using the QI director workforce, which cover all 50 U.S., states plus Puerto Rico. With this support, hospitals are within an environment that drives for success and ease of QI implementation. QI directors are responsible for biannual face-to-face workshops that offer a neutral place for competing hospitals to convene and learn about the latest science and participate in best-practice breakout sessions where they discuss barriers and solutions with other regional hospitals. They are also responsible for regular regional webinars and teleconference calls to continue the momentum gained in workshops and QI multidisciplinary team meetings with hospital staff.

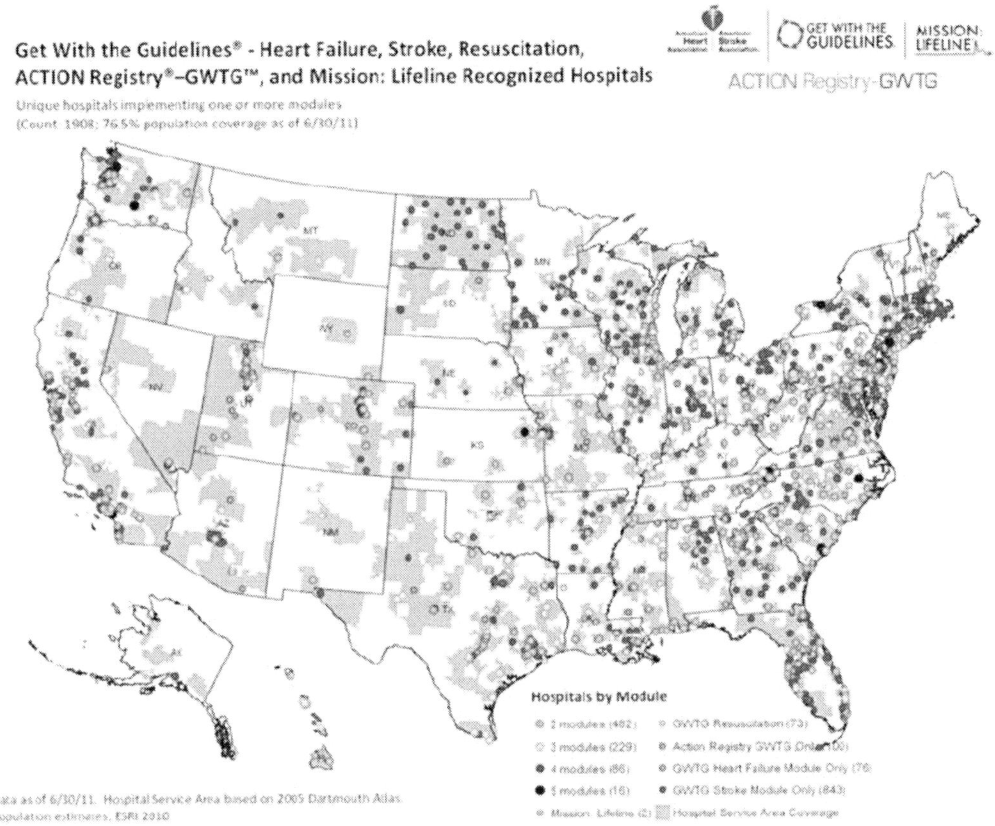

Figure 2. American Heart Association/American Stroke Association on Quality Suite of Programs Recognized Hospitals – U.S. Map.

At the national level, AHA QI staff deploys national QI interventions and advances to support hospital performance improvement. These include national webinars on topics including latest evolving science and guidelines, best practice sharing, program updates, and data collection changes. To provide additional support to local and regional QI efforts, the national AHA team helps to employ the Get With The Guidelines recognition program for each of the different disease-specific modules. To qualify for a Get With The Guidelines Recognition Award, hospitals must reach benchmarks with at least 85% compliance on designated achievement measures for certain time periods (90-days, 12 months, 24 months consecutive or more.) Hospitals that achieve these awards are celebrated at national recognition events including *AHA Scientific Sessions* and/or *AHA/ASA International Stroke Conference.* Hospitals also receive the additional incentive of advertisement celebrating their success in *US News and World Report Top Hospital Edition*, which lists the hospitals according to their recognition status. Starting July 2012, consumers will be able to find these accredited/certified/and award winning AHA/ASA hospitals through the American Heart Association website www.heart.org and www.heart.org/myhealthcare via Google Maps technology. By simply entering a city, state, or zip code consumers (and healthcare providers) will be able to find these hospitals through the click of a mouse.

GET WITH THE GUIDELINES-STROKE

Since 2003, Get With the Guidelines – Stroke is the AHA/ASA's program for continuous QI in hospitals to improve acute stroke treatment and prevent future strokes and cardiovascular events. Stroke, the fourth leading cause of death in the U.S. kills more than 133,000 people annually and is the leading cause of serious long-term disability [1]. On average, every 4 minutes, someone dies of a stroke [2]. Each year, approximately 795,000 people experience a new or recurrent stroke [3]. A patient's outcome depends in large part on timely administration of intravenous thrombolysis (IV rtPA) which has a proven benefit for acute ischemic stroke patients.

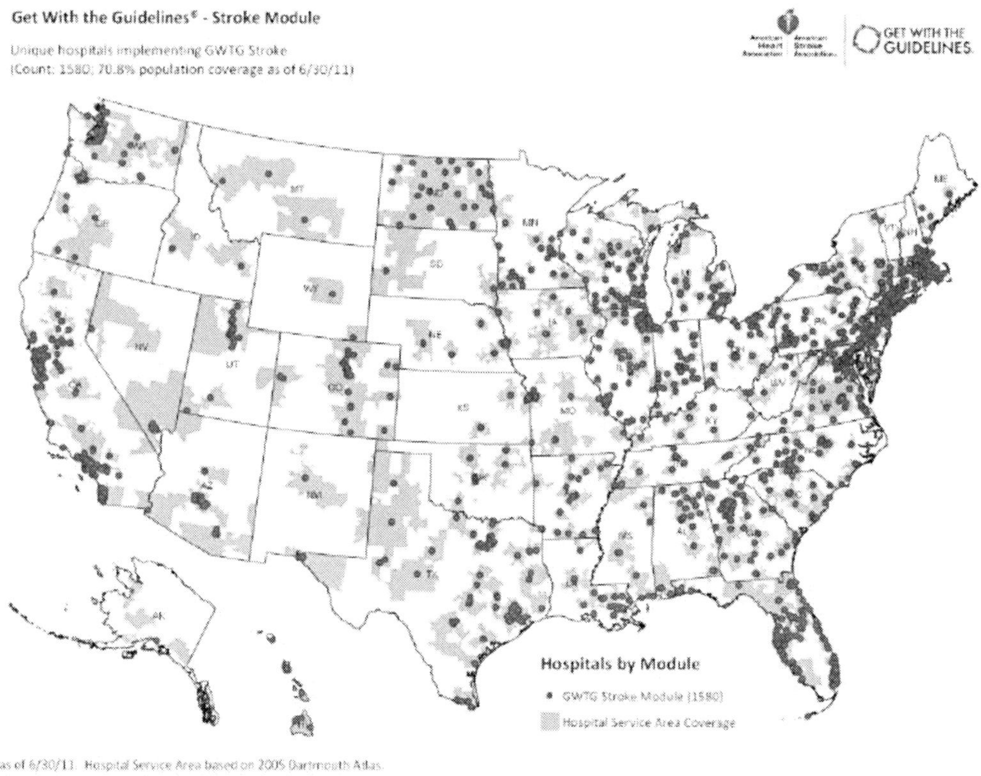

Figure 3. American Heart Association/American Stroke Association Get With The Guidelines-Stroke Map.

Unfortunately, less than one-third of these patients receive IV rtPA within 60 minutes of hospital arrival in the U.S. [4, 5]. Only modest improvement has been seen in the timely administration of IV rtPA in the last 10 years and marked variation in median door-to-needle (DTN) times exist throughout the country [5].

Get With The Guidelines -Stroke focuses on care team protocols to ensure that patients are treated and discharged on appropriate medications and with risk modification counseling. Acute performance measures include use of IV rtPA in patients who arrive in less than 2 hours after symptom onset and treated within 3 hours of symptom onset (acute ischemic strokes only); antithrombotic medication prescribed within 48 hours of admission; deep venous thrombosis prophylaxis; antithrombotic medication at discharge; anticoagulation prescribed at discharge in patients with documented atrial fibrillation; lipid lowering medication prescribed at discharge if LDL > 100 mg/dL; and smoking cessation counseling. Quality measures include initiation of IV rtPA in 60 minutes or less from hospital arrival; dysphagia screening; door-to CT in less than 25 minutes; National Institutes of Health Stroke Scale (NIHSS); stroke education; and patient assessed for and/or received stroke rehabilitation services.

As of June 2012, over 1600 U.S. hospitals were participating in Get With The Guidelines -Stroke with over 2 million patient records entered. The goal is simple: to help hospitals improve outcomes for stroke patients. Progress toward that end is borne out by studies demonstrating improved provision of care over time for hemorrhagic stroke patients at hospitals participating in Get With The Guidelines-Stroke.

In fact, one four-year study of 790 participating hospitals showed a 29-percent increase in the percentage of eligible patients who received IV rtPA within two hours of hospital arrival, a measure that can minimize the extent of damage to the brain and prevent permanent disability. In fact, Get With The Guidelines -Stroke has led to over 40 peer-reviewed manuscripts found in journals such as *Stroke, Circulation, JAHA, Archives of Neurology*, and *American Journal of Cardiology* and multiple podium and poster presentations at International Stroke Conference (ISC), Scientific Sessions, American College of Cardiology Annual Conference (ACC), and Quality Care and Outcomes Research Annual Meeting (QCOR).

Target: Stroke was developed as an extension of Get With The Guidelines -Stroke in early 2010 to specifically focus nationwide efforts in reducing IV rtPA DTN times and further support the information translation and educational needs of healthcare providers caring for this patient population. The goal of Target: Stroke is to achieve DTN times of 60 minutes or less in at least 50% of eligible patients.

Target: Stroke with 1,281 hospitals registered is offered free-of-charge and provides healthcare professionals with *10 Best Practice Strategies* for achieving DTN times of 60 minutes or less for acute ischemic stroke patients.

The strategies are disseminated through protocols, clinical decision support, order sets, guidelines, data measurement tools, feedback processes, and other resources for improving and reporting DTN times. Target: Stroke education leverages multiple media sources, including YouTube, Facebook, Twitter, webinars, local workshops, and in the near-future, a handheld mobile application to reach its target audience.

At its inception in early 2010, 27.7% of patients received IV rtPA in 60 minutes or less. As of December 2011, 24 months after Target: Stroke campaign initiation, 33.4% of patients received IV rtPA in 60 minutes or less. Through the educational effort supported in the course of this proposal we feel confident we can drive this metric close to if not reach our goal of 50%.

Get with the Guidelines-Heart Failure

Get With The Guidelines-Heart Failure, initiated in 2005 with over 500 U.S. hospitals participating is designed to improve the quality of care in patients hospitalized with heart failure. The program aims to help ensure that eligible patients are initiated on guideline recommended therapies and receive appropriate counseling prior to hospital discharge.

Peer-reviewed research (with over 35 manuscripts) has demonstrated that through participating in Get With The Guidelines-Heart Failure, hospitals will provide equitable care (regardless of race, ethnicity, age, or gender), the importance of scheduled physician follow-up after heart failure hospital discharge, the value in device-support as necessary for the acute heart failure patient, and many other significant findings. Our updated Target: Heart Failure is taking a new approach focused on the common factors that contribute to costly re-hospitalizations for patients with heart failure, an area of keen interest and concern for the Centers for Medicare and Medicaid Services (CMS).

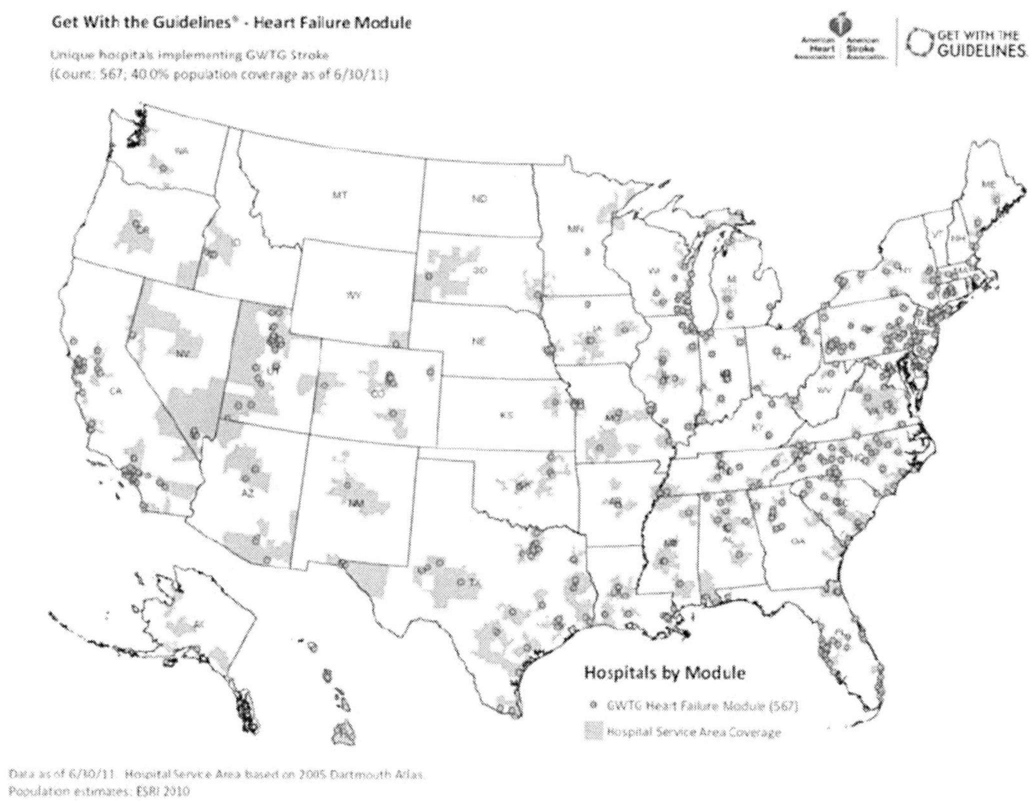

Figure 4. American Heart Association Get With The Guidelines-Heart Failure U.S. Map.

Achievement measures tracked through Get With The Guidelines-Heart Failure and Target: Heart Failure includes:

- Provision of patient-centered HF discharge instructions,
- Measurement of left ventricular (LV) function,

- Prescription for angiotensin-converting enzyme inhibitors (ACE-I) or angiotensin receptor blockers (ARB) and evidence-based beta blocker at discharge provided to patients with left ventricular ejection fraction (LVEF) ≤ .40,
- Prescription for aldosterone antagonist at discharge,
- Counseling for smoking cessation,
- Early post-discharge follow-up with a clinic visit or phone call scheduled to occur within 7 days of discharge, and
- Referral to HF Disease Management, 60 minutes (in-person) patient education, or HF Interactive Workbook.

GET WITH THE GUIDELINES-RESUSCITATION

Get With The Guidelines-Resuscitation formerly the National Registry of Cardiopulmonary Resuscitation (NRCPR) was transitioned in 2011 to promote the QI of inpatient cardiac and respiratory arrest victims including adults, pediatrics, and neonates. As of June 2012, over 290 hospitals have transitioned into/joined the program with 415,000+ patients entered. Similar to Get With the Guidelines-Stroke and Get With The Guidelines-Heart Failure, Get With The Guidelines-Resuscitation also has a vast and deep volume of research generated from the program totaling over 42 manuscripts as of June 2012 found in such journals as *Archives of Internal Medicine, Chest, Resuscitation, Critical Care Medicine, Circulation, Pediatrics, and JAMA* to name a few.

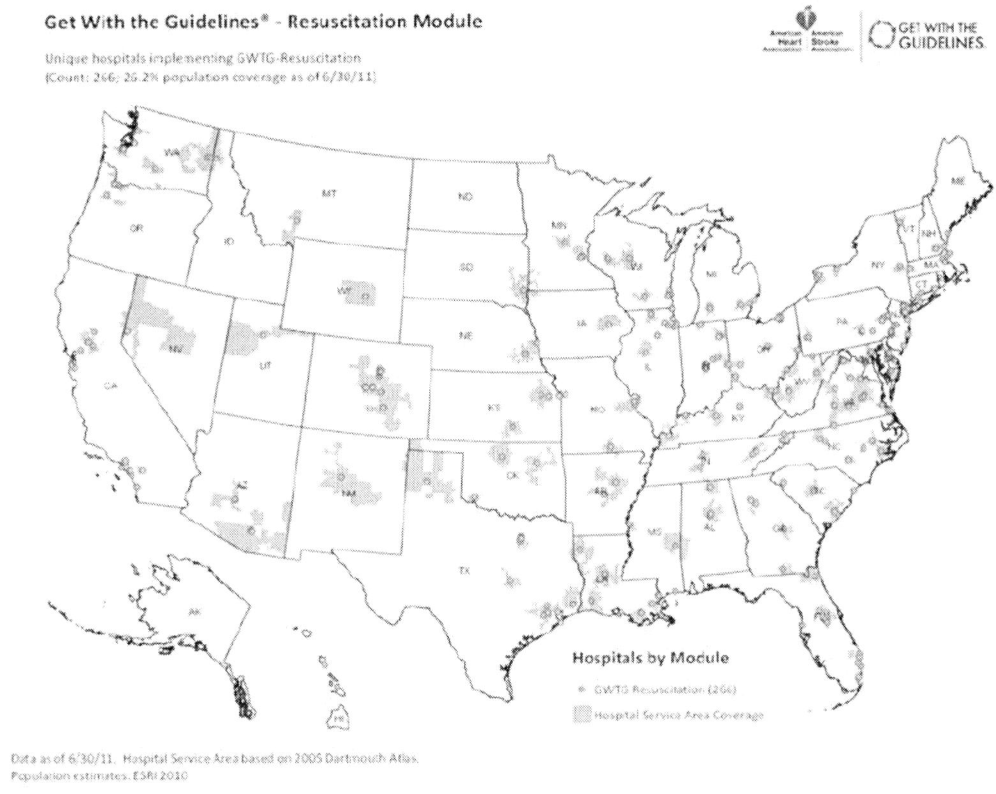

Figure 5. American Heart Association Get With The Guidelines-Resuscitation U.S. Map.

Get with the Guidelines-Stroke, Heart Failure, and Resuscitation Data Flow

Outcome Sciences, Inc. (DBA Outcome) serves as the data collection, repository, and feedback vehicle for hospitals using the Get With The Guidelines-Stroke, Get With The Guidelines-Heart Failure, and Get With The Guidelines-Resuscitation programs.

Hospitals enter into a Participating Hospital Agreement with Outcome, which covers the transmission of patient level data in the form of a limited data set, as defined in the Health Insurance Portability and Accountability Act of 1996. For Get With The Guidelines-Stroke and Get With The Guidelines-Heart Failure, this limited data set is transferred from Outcome to Duke Clinical Research Institute (DCRI) on a quarterly basis under a Data Use Agreement (DUA). The patient level data entered by hospitals is used to provide real-time feedback in the form of reports and guideline checks to facilitate QI and rapid adoption of evidence based guidelines. The Get With The Guidelines volunteer committee provides AHA oversight to Outcome and DCRI. For Get With The Guidelines-Resuscitation, the University of Pennsylvania receives the limited data set from Outcome on a quarterly basis also under a DUA. Similar to Get With The Guidelines -Stroke and Get With The Guidelines -HF, hospitals using Get With The Guidelines-Resuscitation receive real-time feedback reports to facilitate QI and adoption of evidence-based guidelines.

Rigorous data quality measures are taken from more than 1900 hospitals submitting data into the Get With The Guidelines registry. Detailed abstraction guidelines ensure uniform interpretation of information in the medical records across hospitals. Additionally, the Patient Management Tool (PMT) software has real time error and logic checks to provide immediate feedback to users if data values are outside established parameters. Bi-annual quality reports are provided to hospitals to highlight abnormal values and missing or incomplete data. AHA QI staff functions in the role of data support and provide additional training.

DCRI is contracted with the AHA to serve as the data analytic center for Get With The Guidelines. The scope of this agreement is to analyze the aggregate de-identified data for research purposes and program monitoring. Based on the agreed data handling rules, DCRI prepares the dataset for data quality checks, program measure adherence, and for ongoing statistical analyses.

The National Volume Report summarizes the number of records submitted by a specific hospital during the harvest interval, in addition to the total number of records submitted to the modules. This report describes dataset record volume and indicators of data quality, such as the proportion of records excluded, rates of missing data, and descriptive statistics of some of the variables collected.

Mission: Lifeline

Mission: Lifeline is the AHA's national initiative to advance systems of care for patients with ST-segment elevation myocardial infarction (STEMI) by reducing barriers to timely treatment. The overarching goal of the initiative is to reduce mortality and morbidity for STEMI patients and to improve their overall quality of care by reducing systematic delays to treatment.

With the support of Mission: Lifeline, regional programs have been developed to help quickly identify and expedite treatment for STEMI. Mission: Lifeline has been successful in identifying and reducing the system barriers that exist so that care is streamlined. The Mission Lifeline STEMI Systems of care language is now a class I C recommendation in the 2009 ACC/AHA STEMI focused update.

Prior to implementation of Mission: Lifeline in 2007, the National Registry for Myocardial Infarction (NRMI) door to balloon times were 180 minutes.

In 2011, according to data collected in the Action Registry-Get With The Guidelines, 91% of our nation's PCI capable hospitals now achieve door to balloon times in less than 90 minutes. Mortality rates for STEMI patients are directly related to total ischemic time with higher mortality and morbidity associated with longer delays to treatment. STEMI patients who survive delays to treatment may suffer heart failure, decreased ejection fraction and permanent damage to the heart. These patients frequently have longer hospital stays, because of added tests and procedures; all increasing medical expenditures. The Mission: Lifeline initiative is aligned with the AHA's 2020 goals of reducing death and disability from cardiovascular disease and is aligned with our National health care goals of reducing financial burdens associated with chronic disease and disability, which may arise from delays to treatment.

Mission: Lifeline seeks to meet the needs of the patient throughout the continuum of care, beginning with the patient's initial entry into the system (Point of Entry) through each component of the system, and return to the local community and physician for rehabilitative care.

Mission: Lifeline identifies ideal strategies for treatment in the health care system which may begin with EMS, Emergency Department, Referral Centers and those Receiving Centers equipped with 24/7 cardiac catheterization capability.

Get with the Guidelines-Action Registry

In April 2008, the American Heart Association and the American College of Cardiology (ACC) announced the merger of two of the most comprehensive resources for improving quality of care and outcomes for patients with coronary artery disease and acute coronary syndromes resulting in the creation of *ACTION-Registry-Get With The Guidelines.*

The Get With The Guidelines -CAD program closed effective December 31, 2009 with final data entry completed on March 31, 2010. Fiscal year 2010 efforts focused on transitioning Get With The Guidelines -CAD hospitals to ACTION-Registry-GWTG and encouraging Mission: Lifeline hospitals to enroll in ACTION-Registry-GWTG.

Hospitals were encouraged to participate in *ACTION Registry-Get With The Guidelines* with the implementation of various activities including but not limited to:

- Monthly transition webinars for CAD customers co-sponsored by AHA and ACC,
- Informational materials provided to hospitals to encourage Get With The Guidelines -CAD customers to transition and M:L Hospitals to enroll,
- Ongoing education to M:L, QI and State Health Alliance staff via webinar trainings, collateral materials and increased access to AR-G customer website,

- The Limited Form was launched on January 1, 2010 to help reduce data burden on hospitals (see table below),
- Additional certified AR-G vendors allowed more options for hospitals. Certified AR-G vendors now include: NCDR, Outcome Science, Inc., Cedaron, Lumedx, and Heartbase.
- In addition, Lumedx, Cedaron and NCDR began to allow inter-operability between Cath-PCI and AR-G thereby helping to reduce data duplication for hospitals that utilize those vendors for both registries, and,
- The Mission: Lifeline Recognition Program was launched implementing an easier process allowing hospitals to register for M: L as a separate entity thereby creating additional incentives to participate in AR-G.

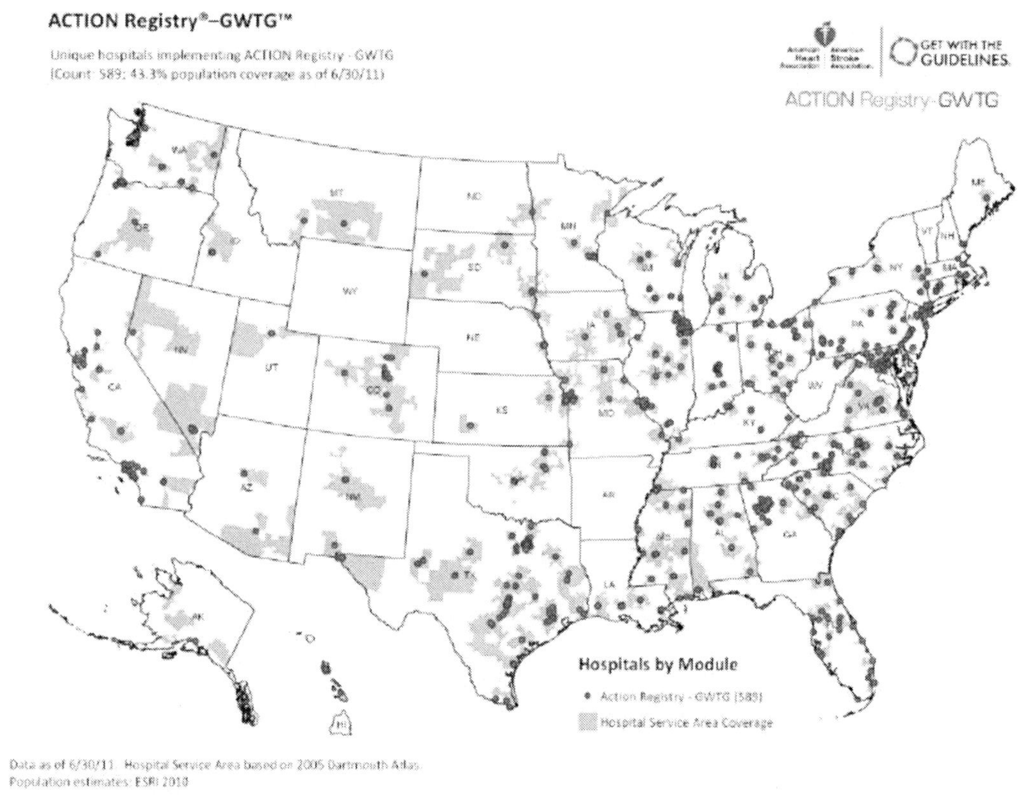

Figure 6. ACTION Registry-GWTG U.S. Map.

The Guideline Advantage

Launched in November 2009, Get With The Guidelines®–Outpatient, was the AHA/ASA's outpatient QI program focused on improving the quality of care delivered by the nearly 150,000 healthcare practices and outpatient clinics nationwide.

This novel program offers practices the opportunity to submit information through their existing electronic health record/health technology platform and, in return, provides feedback reports, which measure treatment to scientific guidelines and benchmark performance achievements. The program is made available to a wide variety of healthcare providers, from general practitioners to cardiovascular specialists, to assess cardiovascular health over time.

In addition, the program offers valuable tools and resources to assist the healthcare provider in their quest for continuous QI. In its initial year, Get With The Guidelines®-Outpatient garnered commitment from 14 electronic health record/health technology companies to offer this program to their nearly 75,000 customers nationwide. Further, this program acts, in part, as measure engine for the American Heart Association's 2020 goal, and aligns with the government's focus on electronic health record adoption.

The Guideline Advantage (formerly Get With The Guidelines-Outpatient) re-launched at the end of March 2011 in collaboration with the American Cancer Society and American Diabetes Association. The program is now a tri-agency initiative that focuses on four of the nation's ten leading causes of death. A new tri-agency staffing and volunteer infrastructure has been established, with AHA taking the operating lead role. Ten practices, representing more than 300 physicians are submitting data into the program in its early phase of development (for more than one million patient records). Electronic health record vendors that have reached the status of Compatible Vendor (meaning they can submit data on behalf of their customers or can enable their customers to participate and they can display the ACS/ADA/AHA Compatible Vendor logo on their marketing materials) include: GEMMS, New Century Health and Forward Health Group. Active discussions continue with other EHR vendors, including.

As of February 2012, The Guideline Advantage began to mirror the "module" approach of Get With The Guidelines as part of an effort to move away from a "one size fits all" approach as different market segments require unique approaches in terms of core measure sets, reports, interventions and recognition. To begin, TGA will focus the components of the program to best suite the distinctive needs of Community Health Centers and Quality Improvement Organizations. The program will continue to have a general approach that would accommodate any site that does not fall into an existing module in an effort to continue growth across the board.

The Guideline Advantage program will continue to offer relevant, clear, credible, concise educational resources and activities that will foster the understanding of chronic disease management and prevention and through education interventions and performance feedback ensuring optimal application in the ambulatory setting. Monthly educational webinars are available to the public; promoted through monthly newsletters, email blasts and the TGA website.

Hospital Accreditation/Certification

In an effort to explore strategic plans, several work groups were formed to brainstorm ideas on how to meet our organizations goals. Out of about 135 work groups-two, different work groups came up with the recommendation to explore hospital recognition.

Because of the work groups efforts and part of the planning process, in August of 2010 the AHA conducted market research with various hospitals and key healthcare professionals across the country. The trends from the interviews were very consistent and positively supported our organization entering into the hospital accreditation space to develop and/or collaborate with external organizations to enhance stroke and cardiac care recognition programs.

As a result of the extensive market research that was completed, we know that hospitals are interested in accreditation or certification primarily to improve the quality of patient care and outcomes they provide their patients and to differentiate them in the market. Our organization's role in hospital accreditation and certification assists hospitals to elevate the quality of patient care provided and ultimately improve the lives of patients with cardiovascular and/or stroke conditions.

With the information gained from the market research, it confirmed that our organization is in a unique position to provide healthcare systems, hospitals, healthcare providers and consumers a nationally recognized accreditation program to distinguish themselves. In December of 2010 an AHA Presidential Advisory was released titled "Hospital Certification for Optimizing Cardiovascular Disease and Stroke Quality of Care and Outcomes" The advisory formally presented our organization's intent to develop and enhance hospital accreditation and certification programs for cardiovascular disease and stroke. Since the advisory was published last December, The Hospital Accreditation initiative has continued to move forward rapidly. Accomplishments include the formation of two volunteer committees to oversee the Hospital Accreditation program, the Hospital Accreditation Business Management Committee and the Hospital Accreditation Science Committee.

The Hospital Accreditation Business Management Committee (that reports to the Corporate Operations Coordinating Committee) and is responsible for the business aspects of Hospital Accreditation.

This Hospital Accreditation business committee has assisted to initiate discussions regarding our role in hospital certification/accreditation with The Joint Commission and the Society of Chest Pain Centers.

The relationship with the Society of Chest Pain Centers is a new relationship for our organization. The Society of Chest Pain Centers is an organization that was founded in 1998 with the mission 'to reduce cardiac deaths' and provides hospitals an operational model of care for acute coronary syndrome patients.

As of December 2011, there are currently 676 certified chest pain centers and 70 additional applications have been received for cycle III certification. By June of 2012, the additional 70 hospitals will be surveyed and will potentially result in over 700 certified chest pain centers by the Society of Chest Pain Centers.

Because our organizations share similar missions, the AHA entered into a business agreement with the Society of Chest Pain Centers (in May of 2011) to provide Mission: Lifeline accreditation for STEMI Referring and Receiving Centers. The goal of the combined effort is to improve the consistency of cardiac care by providing a standard approach to the treatment of STEMI patients. The official launch of the M: L accreditation program was September 2, 2011.

The use of the heart check mark for hospital certification and accreditation programs will allow hospitals to communicate to the patients they serve that they are recognized by the American Heart Association and the American Stroke Association.

The heart check mark is available for use by hospitals that achieve M: L accreditation as a STEMI referral or receiving center. Hospitals that achieve M: L accreditation may use the heart check mark in their marketing materials, patient education materials and consumer and/or community outreach efforts. When the hospital achieves accreditation, it is provided a tool kit of suggested press releases, communications and marketing strategies to assist them to communicate to their patients their accomplishment and that they are a premier provider.

Additionally, we have enhanced our long standing relationship with The Joint (TJC) (since 2003 for Primary Stroke Certification and 2009 for Heart Failure Certification) to offer co-branded programs for Primary Stroke Certification and advanced disease certification for heart failure. The Joint Commission will continue to manage the program, and the AHA/ASA will be responsible for the science framework. This revised relationship will be revenue generating for our organization beginning in 2012.

In addition to the co-branded programs with SCPC and TJC, it is the intent of the Hospital Accreditation program to develop additional accreditation offerings. Existing programs offered by TJC and SCPC have established the building blocks for the AHA and ASA to develop a comprehensive model for cardiac and stroke care.

A Cardiac Task Force has been appointed by the Hospital Accreditation Science Committee and is currently drafting the framework for a new accreditation program, Cardiac Center of Excellence (COE). The Hospital Accreditation Business Committee, with guidance from the Science Committee, will assess and evaluate the options of working either in collaboration with another accrediting body or developing as a standalone AHA offering.

Systems of Care

Currently, throughout health care in the United States, there is a move towards a systems-based approach to care delivery to enhance the efficiency, effectiveness and quality of delivery. This represents a paradigm shift in health care toward team work, standard operating procedures, team accountability and rigorous process adherence to name a few. A systems approach, through the implementation of tools, strategies and standard operating procedures assures that every patient receives the right care at the right time every time. The AHA has been a leader in the introduction of a system's approach to care and has developed a wide variety of systematic approaches across a broad spectrum of clinical areas, including stroke, cardiac arrest and heart failure. In light of this success, an interdivisional team specifically tasked with coordinating, enhancing and facilitating synergy between our various efforts in building high-performing systems (i.e., more efficient, more effective, safer and higher quality). Some of the activities of this group are presented in the next sections.

Quality of Care Outcomes Research Scientific Council

Council Structure

The American Heart Association operates 16 Scientific Councils, such as the Council on Clinical Cardiology (CLCD) and the Council on Quality of Care and Outcomes Research (QCOR), which is an interdisciplinary council with membership that includes physicians, nurses, and health services researchers. It is with the recognition of the essential contribution of the councils to the scientific and administrative goals of the AHA that we recognize the value of the councils and attribute a significant monetary value for the services rendered by the councils in support of the mission of the association to "To build healthier lives, free of cardiovascular diseases and stroke." Council contributions to the AHA mission include:

- Council representatives serve on the national and affiliate research committees and their study sections to peer-review grant applications and determine how to allocate research support each year.
- Council members contribute to the pool of scientists who serve as AHA journal reviewers, editors, and editorial board members.
- Council members are instrumental in determining the nature and scope of professional education activities, including scientific sessions, scientific conferences, and other professional education efforts.
- Council science subcommittees and other council members are responsible for determining at which point knowledge can be incorporated into scientific statements and advisories, and serving on these writing groups. Council members also serve as peer reviewers for AHA scientific statements and science advisories.
- Council members provide input into community-based public education programs offered by AHA affiliates across the country. Council members also assist AHA staff in writing, reviewing, and updating public education materials and portions of the AHA website.
- Additionally, they monitor the state of the art in their disciplines and offer advice and guidance in developing testimony for FDA, NIH, NQF, etc., as well as AHA advocacy efforts.

Specialty Conference

Each May, the QCOR Council sponsors an annual conference on Quality of Care and Outcomes Research in CV Disease and Stroke. This is the pre-eminent meeting of its kind and it is dedicated to the clinical and statistical study of patients' experiences with care. The goal is to leverage these insights to significantly improve the quality of CV and stroke care while actively encouraging informal interaction among attendees and providing networking activities for early career investigators. This conference addresses multiple areas of quality of care, including how to submit grants; patient- and family-centeredness; administering quality patient care; emergency medicine; economics, including value (i.e., cost vs. quality); current national and regional campaigns and initiatives; front line care; nursing research and initiatives; information technology's role in quality of care; health policy; and malpractice. Conference faculty and attendees engage in presentation of cutting-edge research, interactive workshops and "state of the science" learning sessions.

Journal

The QCOR Council is the only AHA scientific council that has an annual specialty conference and a peer-reviewed journal. Circulation: Quality of Care and Outcomes publishes original research contributions-six times per year.

AMERICAN COLLEGE OF CARDIOLOGY/AMERICAN HEART ASSOCIATION TASK FORCES

Clinical Practice Guidelines

Evidence-based clinical documents developed by foremost leaders in the field of cardiology provide a foundation for modern care of patients with cardiovascular disease.-The American Heart Association/American Stroke Association, along with the American College of Cardiology Foundation (ACCF) and other partners, has been developing clinical practice guidelines for more than 20 years.

The guidelines are developed specifically to define strategies for diagnosis and optimal management of cardiovascular disease, including the role of noninvasive and invasive procedures. The Task Force shall also address, when appropriate, the contributions, uniqueness, sensitivity, specificity, indications and contraindications, and cost effectiveness of diagnostic and therapeutic modalities.

Currently there are guidelines for 20 specific conditions or interventions and they are updated on a regular basis. In order to ensure greater responsiveness to the constantly evolving evidence, focused updates are written for specific, timely drugs, devices and best practices.

During this long history, this collaboration has included the development of a rigorous methodology [6, 7]. This methodology was recently highlighted in Appendix D of the recent Institute of Medicine's report on Developing Trustworthy Clinical Practice Guidelines [8]. The ACCF/AHA collaboration on guidelines forms the foundation for the development of performance measure sets [9, 10] that are, when appropriate, drafted in conjunction with the American Medical Association's Physician Consortium for Performance Improvement (AMA PCPI).

The AHA/American Stroke Association also develop clinical practice guidelines for the prevention and management of patients with stroke or trans-ischemic attack.

Performance Measures

Like clinical practice guidelines, the American Heart Association is a leader in creation of measures used for accountability and reimbursement (i.e., Performance Measures) and metrics used for continuous QI, but not accountability (i.e., Quality Metrics). The interest in performance measurement has heightened in recent years given the current environment in medicine, especially the growing national focus on quality.

The joint task force shall develops and promulgates performance measures for the American Heart Association and serves as a source of expertise on performance measurement for the AHA and the American College of Cardiology. This is a listing of some of the activities undertaken by the TF:

- Specify the desirable attributes of performance measures including, but not limited to, measures of structures of care, processes of care, health outcomes, and efficiency;
- Develop statements of principles to guide the development, implementation, revision, and reporting of performance measures;

- Specify an explicit process for the development and maintenance of performance measures that are integrated with the development of ACCF/AHA clinical practice guidelines;
- Develop strategies for creating, testing and maintaining eSpecifications for ACCF/AHA measures to facilitate implementation in Electronic Health Records;
- Partner with other organizations as appropriate in the necessary development, maintenance, and field testing of performance measures in high-priority clinical areas;
- As necessary, review and comment on measures developed by other organizations that are relevant to the guidelines, scientific statements and expert consensus documents of the ACC and AHA;
- As necessary, formulate an educational strategy about performance measurement; and integration into electronic health registries/systems.
- Serve as a source of expertise and advice to the ACC and AHA regarding performance measurement.

Because the performance measures are typically guideline-based, usually requiring a Class I level of recommendation (i.e., should be done) there existed a need for a new methodology for advanced technologies used in diagnosis and treatment of CV disease, such as cardiac imaging, for which there are often no underlying guideline documents. Because these technologies affect the quality of cardiovascular care and have the potential to contribute to cardiovascular health expenditures, there is a need for more critical assessment of the use of technology, including the development of quality and performance measures in areas in which guideline recommendations are absent [11].

Data Standards

Another burgeoning field is the development of clinical data standards that provide uniform language to describe the evaluation, treatment, and outcomes of patients with a range of cardiovascular conditions and serve as a source of expertise on clinical data standards for the American Heart Association.

Here are some of the activities that the Task Force carries out:

- Specify and define, as appropriate, the data elements and corresponding definitions to be used in describing patient clinical management and outcomes, for research, in epidemiological assessments and for use in clinical registries and cardiovascular disease-related professional documents (e.g., guidelines and performance measures);
- Define the methodology to guide the development and ongoing maintenance of clinical data standards;
- Develop explicit strategies and processes to promote ongoing harmonization of clinical data standards across all AHA clinical documents and initiatives;
- Optimize opportunities for sharing data across various sources in order to promote optimal cardiovascular care and disease prevention;
- Collaborate with other organizations and with internal ACC and AHA committees, including the ACC/AHA Task Force on Performance Measures, the ACCF/AHA

Task Force on Practice Guidelines, and the AHA Get With The Guidelines Steering Committee, as appropriate, in the development, maintenance, and promotion of clinical data standards;
- Identify strategies to promote and implement ACC/AHA clinical data standards in a variety of environments including, but not limited to, electronic health records.

REFERENCES

[1] Roger VL, Go As, Lloyd-Jones DM, Adams RJ, Berry, JD, Brown TM et al. AHA statistical update: Heart disease and stroke statistics 2011 update: A report from the American Heart Association. *Circulation* 2011, 123: e18-e209.

[2] Centers for Disease Control and Prevention. Vital statistics public use data files – 2008 Mortality multiple cause files. Available at http:// www.cdc.gov/nchs/data-_access/vitalstatsonline.htm#mortality_ multiple. Accessed September 23, 2011.

[3] Roger VL, Go AS, Lloyd-Jones DM, Benjamin EJ, Berry JD, Bordon WB et al. Heart disease and stroke statistics 2012 update: a report from the American Heart Association. *Circulation* 2012; 124: e2-e220.

[4] Fonarow CG, Smith EE, Saver JL, Reeves MJ, Bhatt DL, Grau-Sepulveda MV, et al. Timeliness of tissue-type plasminogen activator therapy in acute ischemic stroke: Patient characteristics, hospital factors, and outcomes association with door-to-needle times within 60 minutes. *Circulation* 2011; 123: 750-758.

[5] Fonarow GC, Smith EE, Saver JL, Reeves MJ, Hernandez AF, Peterson ED et al. Improving door-to-needle times in acute ischemic stroke. The design and rationale for the American Heart Association/American Stroke Association's Target: Stroke initiative. *Stroke* 2011: 42:2983-2989.

[6] Gibbons RJ, Smith S, Antman EM. The American College of Cardiology/American Heart Association Clinical Practice Guidelines: Part I: Where Do They Come From? *Circulation.* 2003;107:2979–2986.

[7] Gibbons RJ, Smith, Jr, SC; Antman EM. American College of Cardiology/American Heart Association Clinical Practice Guidelines: Part II: Evolutionary Changes in a Continuous Quality Improvement Project. *Circulation.* 2003;107:3101-3107.

[8] IOM (Institute of Medicine). 2011. *Clinical Practice Guidelines We Can Trust.* Washington, DC: The National Academies Press.

[9] Spertus JA, Eagle KA, Krumholz HM, Mitchell KR, Normand ST. ACC/AHA methodology for the selection and creation of performance measures for quantifying the quality of cardiovascular care: a report of the ACC/AHA Task Force on Performance Measures. *Circulation* 2005; 111:1703–1712.

[10] Spertus JA, Bonow RO, Chan P, Diamond GA, Drozda JP Jr, Kaul S, Krumholz HM, Masoudi FA, Normand S-LT, Peterson ED, Radford MJ, Rumsfeld JS. ACCF/AHA new insights into the methodology of performance measurement: a report of the American College of Cardiology Foundation/American Heart Association Task Force on Performance Measures. *Circulation.* 2010;122:2091–2106.

[11] Bonow RO, Douglas PS, Buxton AE, Cohen DJ, Curtis JP, DeLong E, Drozda JP Jr, Ferguson TB Jr, Heidenreich PA, Hendel RC, Masoudi FA, Peterson ED, Taylor AJ. ACCF/AHA methodology for the development of quality measures for cardiovascular technology: a report of the American College of Cardiology Foundation/American

Heart Association Task Force on Performance Measures. *Circulation.* 2011; 124:1483–1502.

In: Quality Improvement
Editors: K. W. Lobdell and S. C. Stamou
ISBN: 978-1-62417-390-5

Chapter 2

THE GERMAN EXPERIENCE WITH INDICATOR-BASED QUALITY IMPROVEMENT

***Peter C. Scriba*[1]*, Ulrike Nimptsch*[2] *and Thomas Mansky*[2,*]**
[1]Scientific Board of the Federal Chamber of Physicians (Bundesärztekammer), Berlin, Germany
[2]Department for Structural Advancement and Quality Management in Healthcare, Technische Universität Berlin, Berlin, Germany

ABSTRACT

Considerable progress has been made in quality assessment in German hospitals over the last decade. Parallel to the advancement of mandatory quality measures based on a separate system of data collection, the development of quality indicators derived from hospital discharge data has become possible with the availability of this administrative data.

This chapter illustrates recent advancements of the German Inpatient Quality Indicators (G-IQI), their current application for quality improvement in German acute care hospitals, and their potential application in monitoring quality of care at the national level.

INTRODUCTION

German hospitals are legally bound to participate in a mandatory quality assurance system, which involves quality measurement for specific diseases and hospital services. This mandatory quality assurance system is based on data which is collected separately, in addition to administrative data collected in the process of daily hospital operations, and serves as a nationwide benchmarking exercise.

It is currently being extended to ambulatory specialist and primary care settings, whereby healthcare delivery across different sectors will be captured (Szecsenyi et al. 2012).

---

[*] E-mail addresses: peter.scriba@med.uni-muenchen.de, thomas.mansky@tu-berlin.de.

Additionally, German hospitals are obliged to maintain an internal quality management system and to report on their activities via hospital quality reports. Providers are allowed free choice with regard to this internal quality management strategy.

In terms of quality improvement, measurement of quality indicators is the prerequisite for identification of potential problems in the process of care, and for monitoring the effectiveness of improvement activities. Since the collection of separate data for quality measurement demands considerable documentation effort of physicians, nurses and other healthcare specialists, use of existing administrative data presents significant advantages – as far as such data is available and reliable.

In Germany, the introduction of a reimbursement system for inpatient services based on Diagnosis Related Groups (DRG) provided the foundation of quality measurement based on administrative data. From 2003 onward, this type of reimbursement has been applicable to all inpatient services (except psychiatry) in acute care hospitals. In Germany, the system includes all patients and all payers - consequently, all inpatient episodes are being recorded electronically in a standardized form. The format of German DRG data is widely comparable to those of other health care systems utilizing DRGs for hospital reimbursement purposes; this includes demographic information, principal and secondary diagnoses, hours of mechanical ventilation, length of stay, admission mode and discharge disposition, among other information.

Coding of diagnoses and procedures in Germany did not begin with the introduction of the DRG system, but this change brought with it an important improvement in data quality. Documentation of diagnoses based on ICD-9 was introduced in 1986, and updated to ICD-10 in 2000. Procedure coding based on ICPM (the 'International Classification of Procedures in Medicine' - the widely extended and modernized German version is named OPS) became mandatory in 1995.

However, prior to 2003, the quality of coding was inconsistent due to the lack of incentives and consequences. Introduction of the DRG system was accompanied by the implementation of strict coding guidelines and regulations for controlling the quality of coding. As a result, the quality of administrative data available from German hospital information systems improved significantly (Busse et al. 2009).

The availability of reliable data drove the development of voluntary indicator-based quality improvement initiatives in Germany. The following sections will describe the indicators used, the application of improvement strategies in German hospitals, and related perspectives of health services research.

QUALITY MEASUREMENT BASED ON ADMINISTRATIVE DATA IN GERMANY

The Helios hospital group – a for-profit provider of hospital services in Germany – were the pioneers in the use of administrative data for the purpose of quality management. In 2000 the group began to develop an outcome-driven quality management system for acute care hospital services, which was based on three core aspects: Monitoring quality indicators derived from administrative data, public reporting of results, and peer review procedures.

Table 1. German Inpatient Quality Indicators, Version 3.1: Overview of included diseases and procedures

No	Disease / procedure
1	Acute myocardial infarction
2	Heart failure
3	Left heart catheterization
4	Cardiac arrhythmia
5	Pacemakers and implantable defibrillators
6	Cardiac ablation
7	Heart surgery
8	Stroke
9	TIA (transient ischemic attack)
10	Early geriatric rehabilitation
11	Pneumonia
12	Chronic obstructive pulmonary disease
13	Lung cancer
14	Thoracic surgery
15	Cholecystectomy
16	Herniotomy
17	Thyroid resection
18	Colorectal resection
19	Gastric resection
20	Oesophageal resection
21	Pancreatic resection
22	Carotid procedures
23	Aortic aneurysm procedures
24	Lower limb arterial occlusive disease procedures
25	Amputation
26	PTA of the lower limb
27	Delivery
28	Newborns
29	Hysterectomy
30	Breast cancer
31	Mastectomy
32	Hip replacement (primary)
33	Hip replacement (revision)
34	Knee replacement (primary)
35	Knee replacement (revision)
36	Hip or knee replacement for neoplasm
37	Spine surgery
38	Hip fracture
39	Polytrauma
40	Nephrectomy
41	Cystectomy
42	Transurethral resection (TUR) of the prostate
43	Radical prostatectomy
44	Kidney stones
45	Multi organ procedures
46	Mechanical ventilation
47	Septicemia
48	Autopsy rate

Inspired by the AHRQ Inpatient Quality Indicators, the Helios quality indicator set mainly focussed on volumes and inpatient mortality for relevant diseases and major procedures. Over more than 10 years, a continued, iterative process of defining, applying, discussing and redefining these measures has been undertaken, supported by clinicians of the Helios hospitals. This has led to a sophisticated set of indicators, which currently is much more detailed than the AHRQ indicators.

Since 2010 the advancement of this indicator set is being continued at the Berlin Institute of Technology (Technische Universität Berlin). The technical specifications of the indicator set, now called 'German Inpatient Quality Indicators' (G-IQI), are freely accessible (Mansky et al. 2011). The G-IQI system is currently used by approximately 500 German hospitals of all kinds of ownership. The national quality indicator systems in Switzerland (BAG 2012) and Austria (Fuchs et al. 2010) are also based on G-IQI. Ongoing refinement is primarily driven by the input of clinicians, who are utilizing the measures in their everyday clinical work.

In its current version 3.1, the G-IQI set covers diseases and procedures that are also included in the IQI system developed by AHRQ, such as acute myocardial infarction, heart failure, stroke, pneumonia, and cholecystectomy. However, the G-IQI set is even more differentiated and comprehensive, covering almost 39% of all German inpatient episodes (Nimptsch and Mansky 2012). Table 1 displays an overview of the diseases and procedures covered by the current G-IQI set. Volume indicators are given for all diseases. Mortality and other outcome indicators are added, wherever they make sense and are feasible.

A modified version of such indicators can also be used for the analysis of long term data from insurance companies. This extends the scope of outcome measurement beyond the inpatient stay and enables the measurement of long term indicators. Insurance data contain a unique personal identifier, which allows us to link a start event, such as a hospitalization for AMI or a total hip replacement, for example, with subsequent information on mortality after 30 or 90 days. Further, readmissions or surgery for complications can be followed, even if the patient was readmitted to a different hospital.

The largest group of German sickness funds – AOK - developed such a set of long-term indicators in cooperation with the Scientific Institute of the AOK, the research institute FEISA (Forschungs- und Entwicklungsinstitut für das Sozial- und Gesundheitswesen Sachsen-Anhalt) and the Helios hospital group (AOK-Bundesverband et al. 2007). This indicator set is called QSR. The further advancement of the QSR indicators is being conducted by the Scientific Institute of the AOK. All German hospitals can request QSR measures, based on the data of their AOK-insured patients. These measures are provided by the AOK via annual reports.

Application of Indicator-Based Quality Improvement Strategies in Hospitals

Outcome measurement is an important requisite for quality improvement, but the story does not end there. It is also essential that these measures be delivered in a timely manner in order to identify abnormal results within a practically appropriate timeframe. This may also lead into auditing of patient records and peer review procedures for critical cases, which is a process with the potential to identify areas for improvement.

The effectiveness of such improvement activities can then be monitored via periodic measurement of the indicators, which closes the loop of the continuous quality improvement circle.

Such an approach has been applied by the Helios hospitals, who were at the forefront of the implementation of this quality improvement strategy. This approach has led to remarkable reductions of inpatient mortality for important diseases, such as AMI, heart failure, pneumonia and stroke (Busse et al. 2009, Krahwinkel et al. 2010).

In 2008 the 'Initiative Qualitätsmedizin' (initiative for quality in medical care, IQM) was funded by 14 hospital providers of all kinds of ownership. IQM is a voluntary non-profit association of hospitals committed to a quality strategy based on three principles:

- Measuring quality indicators based on administrative data,
- transparency by public reporting, and
- peer review procedures to identify weaknesses in the treatment process (which then become the focus of improvement initiatives).

The quality indicators as used by IQM rely on G-IQI, but QSR indicators are also used for long-term information. IQM provides a platform for exchange of know-how, and for 'learning from the best' via cooperative support, e.g. due to conducting cross-hospital peer reviews. As of 2012, approximately 200 hospitals in Germany, Austria and Switzerland are members of IQM, treating more than 3.5 million patients per year (Initiative Qualitätsmedizin 2012).

The peer review procedures are a crucial element of quality improvement: they address potential problems in areas of guideline adherence, interdisciplinary cooperation, cross-departmental processes or infrastructure.

Interpretation of possible errors or deficiencies and their causes requires involvement of medical experts who are capable of discourse with senior physicians at the same level (peers) in a collegial atmosphere (Flintrop and Gerst 2011). For this reason, peer reviews performed within IQM are based on the following principles:

- All peers are senior physicians themselves,
- Colleague-to-colleague suggestions (eye-to-eye),
- open culture for handling errors,
- learning from errors and learning from each other, and
- external support is made available to all.

When out-of-norm results are identified via the quality indicators, a peer review team consisting of three senior physicians from three different IQM member hospitals visit their colleague at the site in question to undertake the review together, as peers. Besides their medical expertise, all peers are trained for the appraisal of critical cases. The review is conducted by analyzing patient records of critical cases retrospectively. Based on the findings of the review, conclusions are drawn for future changes and improvement activities. (Rink 2011, Rink and Eberlein-Gonska 2010). Since the early days, the IQM peer review procedures have been supported by the German Federal Chamber of Physicians (Bundesärztekammer), who have developed a curriculum for educating physicians as peer reviewers (Chop 2011).

Quality Indicators and Health Services Research

Since the German DRG reimbursement system for hospital services covers all acute care hospitals and all types of insurance, the DRG data represent a complete all-patient/all-payer database of hospital care in Germany. The entire German DRG database is accessible via the German Federal Statistical Office for scientific research purposes.

Within a recently finalized study based on this national data, the indicators of G-IQI were used to analyze characteristics of inpatient care in German hospitals (Nimptsch and Mansky 2012). The analysis provides an overview of total national case numbers, numbers of hospitals providing certain inpatient services, the national inpatient mortality, and further indicators of the G-IQI set. Volume indicators were derived from quartiles of case number per hospital. Quartiles of mortality per hospital were calculated to assess outcome on the hospital level.

The results of this analysis provide national reference values for those hospitals which apply G-IQI in their quality management. This is highly valuable for the self-assessment of a hospital's position relative to the German average. For this purpose, all national reference values will be published in the upcoming version of the G-IQI technical specification.

Furthermore, the analysis revealed some potential structural problems in Germany. For example, for uncommon diseases and procedures that are performed less frequently, such as oesophageal resection or cystectomy, very low volumes were observed in the low-volume quartile of hospitals. Assuming a volume-outcome relationship for such complex interventions (Birkmeyer et al. 2002), quality improvements on the national level might be achievable if structural problems were to be addressed. In the case of pancreatic resection, for example, the lower quartile of the 748 hospitals performing this procedure in 2010 performed only 1 or 2 operations per year (Nimptsch and Mansky 2012). A further concentration of such procedures seems to be advisable.

The national DRG data is an important resource for health services research in Germany. It can be used for evaluations of the effectiveness of quality improvement strategies, as applied by IQM, in comparison to national trends. Since the data format is comparable to that of many other countries it can also be used for international comparisons of quality in healthcare.

Conclusion

In Germany, the development of quality assessment based on administrative data has been driven by data availability since the introduction of the DRG system. The G-IQI indicator set described in this chapter is used on a voluntary basis in Germany. The mandatory quality assurance system also intends to utilize administrative data in future (Szecsenyi et al. 2012).

Voluntary quality improvement strategies based on outcome indicators are gaining more and more acceptance and popularity in Germany. On a national level, such strategies are also being introduced to varied extent in Switzerland and Austria: the Swiss adoption will focus on public reporting, while Austria attempts an introduction of the indicators in combination with peer reviews.

Current experiences with indicator-based quality improvement strategies, such as in the Helios hospital group, are promising: strong improvement effects were seen for those hospitals initially performing below par (publication pending). The effectiveness of such approaches on patient outcomes in other settings will be subject to future research.

REFERENCES

AOK-Bundesverband, Forschungs- und Entwicklungsinstitut für das Sozial- und Gesundheitswesen Sachsen-Anhalt (FEISA), HELIOS Kliniken, Wissenschaftliches Institut der AOK (WIdO), *Qualitätssicherung der stationären Versorgung mit Routinedaten (QSR) – Abschlussbericht,* WIdO, Bonn (2007).

Birkmeyer JD, Siewers AE, Finlayson EV, Stukel TA, Lucas FL, Batista I, Welch HG, Wennberg DE, Hospital volume and surgical mortality in the United States. *N. Engl. J. Med.* 346, 1128-37 (2002).

Bundesamt für Gesundheit (Ed.), *Qualitätsindikatoren der Schweizer Akutspitäler 2008/2009,* Bundesamt für Gesundheit, Bern (2012).

Busse R, Nimptsch U, Mansky T, Measuring, Monitoring, and Managing Quality in Germany's Hospitals. *Health Affairs* 28, w294-w304 (2009).

Chop I, Was Peers noch lernen können. Von der Evaluation der IQM-Reviews zum Curriculum Ärztliches Peer Review der Bundesärztekammer. In: Kuhlen R, O Rink, J Zacher (Eds.) *Jahrbuch Qualitätsmedizin 2011,* MVV, Berlin 129-38 (2011).

Fuchs F, Amon M, Nimptsch U, Mansky T, *A-IQI | Austrian Inpatient Quality Indicators,* Universitätsverlag der TU Berlin, Berlin (2010). http://opus. kobv.de/tuberlin/volltexte/2010/2722/.

Initiative Qualitätsmedizin. Routinedaten, Transparenz, Peer Review – für die bestmögliche medizinische Behandlungsqualität [website] http://www. initiative-qualitaetsmedizin.de/home/ (June 20th 2012).

Krahwinkel W, Rink O, Liebetrau M, Günther M, Schuler E, Kuhlen R, [10 years of Peer Reviewing - improving treatment by quality indicators from administrative data.] *Dtsch. Med. Wochenschr.* 136, 2083-8 (2011).

Mansky T, Nimptsch U, Winklmair C, Vogel K, Hellerhoff F, *G-IQI | German Inpatient Quality Indicators Version 3.1,* Universitätsverlag der TU Berlin, Berlin (2011). http://opus.kobv.de/tuberlin/volltexte/2011/3004/.

Nimptsch U, Mansky T, [Disease-specific patterns of hospital care in Germany analyzed via the German Inpatient Quality Indicators (G-IQI)] *Dtsch. Med. Wochenschr.* 137, 1449-57 (2012).

Rink O, Eberlein-Gonska M, Peer Review – wie wir Qualität verbessern lernen. In: Kuhlen R, Rink O, Zacher J (Eds.) *Jahrbuch Qualitätsmedizin 2010,* MVV, Berlin 59-70 (2010).

Rink O, Peer Review im Krankenhaus: Evaluation zeigt: Es gibt noch Verbesserungspotenzial. *Deutsches Ärzteblatt* 108, A1518-20 (2011).

Szecsenyi J, Broge B, Eckhardt J, Heller G, Kaufmann-Kolle P, Wensing M, Tearing down walls: opening the border between hospital and ambulatory care for quality improvement in Germany. *Int. J. Qual. Health Care* 24, 101-4 (2012).

SECTION TWO: EDUCATION

In: Quality Improvement
Editors: K. W. Lobdell and S. C. Stamou
ISBN: 978-1-62417-390-5

Chapter 3

QUALITY IMPROVEMENT EDUCATION: A TOOL FOR TRANSFORMATION OF HEALTHCARE

***Laura Noonan*[1], *Cheryl Courtlandt*[2], *Maureen Walsh Koricke*[3], *Sarah Mabus*[3] *and Leonard Feld*[4]**

[1]Director, Center for Advancing Pediatric Excellence, Department of Pediatrics, Levine Children's Hospital at Carolinas Medical Center,Charlotte Area Health Education Center, Carolinas HealthCare System, Charlotte, NC, US
[2]Co-Director, Center for Advancing Pediatric Excellence, Pediatric Asthma Program and Attending, Department of Pediatrics, Levine Children's Hospital at Carolinas Medical Center, Carolinas HealthCare System, Charlotte, NC, US
[3]Center for Advancing Pediatric Excellence, Department of Pediatrics, Levine Children's Hospital at Carolinas Medical Center, Carolinas HealthCare System, Charlotte, NC, US
[4]Levine Children's Hospital, Sara H. Bissell and Howard C. Bissell Endowed Chair in Pediatrics, Department of Pediatrics, Chief Medical Officer, Levine Children's Hospital at Carolinas Medical Center, Carolinas HealthCare System, Charlotte, NC, US

ABSTRACT

The healthcare industry and medical clinicians have been slow to embrace proven quality improvement (QI) methods to improve outcomes and promote patient safety.

Industries with outstanding safety profiles and predictable outcomes have incorporated these methods into daily operations and have reaped the benefits of decreased variability, decreased error, and increased cost-savings.

In a healthcare setting, QI has the potential to radically alter the quality of care provided to both individual patients and entire patient populations. Demonstration of QI skills is increasingly being required of healthcare staff at all stages of education and practice.

The need for acquisition of these skills has challenged educators and educational institutions to develop new approaches to incorporate learning and practicing QI skills into their medical curriculum. In order to decrease waste and improve patient safety, all levels of medical training must include mastery of these QI methods to achieve desired outcomes and to improve the efficiency and effectiveness of the healthcare delivered.

This chapter spotlights an innovative approach to QI education, a longitudinal progressive 3-year resident curriculum developed by the Center for Advancing Pediatric Excellence (CAPE)in the Department of Pediatrics at Carolinas Medical Center in Charlotte, North Carolina. Based on adult learning theory, the curriculum utilizes self-directed, experiential and transformational learning techniques. The CAPE QI curriculum is rooted in individualized coaching which rigorously pairs knowledge transfer with active hands-on training. A stepped, progressive hands-on curriculum further entrenches QI skills by establishing fundamentals and building on previous experience. This resident curriculum culminates in a leadership experience that hardwires learned QI skills into future practice.

QI education that is integrated into a medical curriculum on both the graduate and undergraduate level has the potential to transform the delivery of medical care. This transformation can improve outcomes, eliminate waste, improve efficiency, foster teamwork and increase patient safety.

The necessary skills can be incorporated into medical curriculums assuring that medical providers of the future deliver patient-centered quality healthcare.

Providers currently in practice who have not received training in QI will require education as the entire healthcare delivery system is being revamped to reward desirable outcomes.

INTRODUCTION

In 1910, Abraham Flexner and the Carnegie Foundation for the Advancement of Teaching engaged in an extensive study of all existing medical schools in the United States and Canada, examining entrance requirements and curriculum, type of medicine taught, quality and quantity of teaching faculty, institutional financial status and available clinical resources. The results of his work, called the Flexner Report [1] revolutionized the approach to the evaluation of medical education. One result of the Flexner Report in conjunction with initiatives by the American Medical Association, wasto base medical education in research-based medical universities. [2] Flexner noted, "We have indeed in America medical practitioners not inferior to the best elsewhere; but there is probably no other country in the world in which there is so great a distance and so fatal a difference between the best, the average, and the worst." Quality and consistency in medical education in United States and Canada was divergent and dangerous. Students with affluence or greater insight sought additional training in Europe due to the increased rigor of their clinical and laboratory curriculum to address deficits in their medical education.

Both undergraduate and graduate medical education have made significant strides in the improvement of medical education within the Flexnerian model. Today most medical schools and residency programs have embraced technology and new teaching methods and have incorporated into their curriculum web-based learning resources, leveraged technology using simulations, and utilized standardized patients for instruction and clinical assessment. As a result of efforts of the Accreditation Council on Graduate Medical Education (ACGME) [3], there are clearly defined learning objectives and competencies. New teaching methods utilize small groups and case studies for more in depth practice-based education.

These efforts at innovation in medical education are worthy of praise but medical care has become so complex and fragmented that medical quality of care has decreased and medical errors have increased to unacceptable rates. Over the last 10 years, there has been increasing attention to improving the quality of care delivered to patients and patient safety. According to the Institute of Medicine (IOM) [4] medical care should be safe, effective, patient-centered, timely, efficient and equitable. Medical education must be transformed to meet these goals. Both the ACGME and the Association of American Medical Colleges (AAMC) have been examining the role of medical education in producing a medical workforce that provides competent and compassionate care in an effective and efficient manner. Both organizations have implemented policies for undergraduate and graduate medical education focused on developing these competencies. AAMC has mandated that quality improvement and patient safety be incorporated into undergraduate medical education and on the graduate level the ACGME has established competencies in practice-based learning and improvement and systems-based practice[3]. Certifying bodies support this philosophy, as demonstrated by the Accreditation Council for Continuing Medical Education (ACCME) [5] requiring a QI component in order to obtain the highest level of accreditation.

With these issues in mind, a 2010 analysis of medical education both on the undergraduate and graduate level using similar methodology as the Flexner Report was undertaken. The findings suggest that medical students experience inflexible training that is not student-centered and there is a persistence of some archaic teaching models not based on current models of best practice for adult learning. Numerous conflicts were revealed in the balance between inpatient and outpatient exposure, institutional service needs, faculty support for the mission of teaching and overarching concerns of institutions with dwindling reimbursement and overall economic recession. The study also revealed commercial interest is directing the allocation of resources and the practice of medicine [6].

Further examination of current medical training shows that trainees have limited experiences that connect knowledge and skills, one of the primary tenets of adult learning theory. Little attention has been paid to population-based care, outcomes, or effectiveness of care. Sophisticated technologies are enhancing diagnostic capabilities and expanding options for extending the life span. At the same time quality health care is not accessible to all in the United States. Instilling QI in medical education is a necessity to manage costs, achieve better outcomes and deliver a consistent high level of quality of medical care. Medical schools and residency training programs are a logical time to introduce and integrate QI skills with clinical skills as training progresses. With appropriate training, medical students and residents can develop the necessary skills to become active participants in QI and progress into leadership positions on QI teams.

Residency is an ideal opportunity to initiate and embed QI into physicians' daily practice. Residents are constantly learning and integrating new information into their work. As front-line providers, they are intimately involved with patient care and able to navigate across discipline and staff boundaries. QI is the quintessential team sport, reliant on collaboration amongst a broad range of staff that fulfills specifically assigned QI team roles. Basing QI education in a residency training program has the added benefit of extending the spread to other programs, institutions, or physician practices.

This education and training must also be implemented with providers who are already practicing in the field. In addition to including QI education in medical school and residency programs, a systematic approach is necessary to formally educate physicians who graduated before QI was mandated in training programs.

Quality Improvement Methods

QI methods have an early history in manufacturing and production. Juran [7], Demming [8] and Shewhart [9] made major contributions in the use of statistical process control methods to reduce variation, eliminate waste and consequently reduce cost. These methods used in industry since the 1930's are fairly new to healthcare. There are many widely used methodologies within improvement science, such as Lean [10], Six Sigma [11], Lean-Six Sigma [12], and the Model for Improvement [13]. All of these methods have some applicability to various areas in healthcare delivery. These QI methods have similar goals of error reduction, minimizing unnecessary variation, decreasing waste, maximizing value, and improving outcomes.

Lean production, derived from Japanese manufacturing techniques, was introduced by Krafcik, a quality engineer at Toyota, as a quality improvement methodology that seeks to improve processes by elimination of waste and promoting the concept of value. Fundamental elements of this method are understanding the concept of value and what constitutes value to the customer or consumer and understanding waste and its relationship to the process being studied.

A series of principles such as Root Cause Analysis and 5 Whys can be utilized to understand both value and waste within a process. Another Lean efficiency principle, called 5S, incorporates standardization to organize objects and supplies. The five S's are sort, set in order, shine, standardize and sustain. These operational tenets are implemented to maintain organization, aid in visual identification, and promote cleanliness. This method, often applied in large corporations, can enable standardization and organization can be realized throughout an enterprise even world wide. This concept allows any employee to function in diverse settings. The 5S method has been adapted to healthcare settings since clinicians may move frequently between multiple complex settings in the course of a day and waste time looking for objects necessary to complete tasks. Numerous hospitals have incorporated Lean methodology to organize and standardize inpatient services, especially operating room services.

Six Sigma [11] is a business strategy, developed at Motorola for process improvement that focuses on improving quality by identifying errors or variation of process in order to decrease variation, remove error, and decrease cost.

This method uses statistical process to control variability and decrease errors as well as personnel that are specially trained. It is disseminated in organizations by masters who have belts (black, brown, yellow) that describe their experience with this problem-solving methodology. Precise specifications are set for processes, outcomes and performance.

Recently, some of the ideas of Six Sigma and Lean manufacturing have been combined to create a new methodology named Lean-Six Sigma [12]. The Lean-Six Sigma methodology takes Lean principles that examine work flow, process and waste and align these principles with Six Sigma, which focuses on control of variation and reduction of error. Further details for quality improvement methods and tools can be obtained from references.

Finally, the quality improvement method The Model for Improvement [13], published by Associates in Process Improvement (API), is the method utilized by the Institute for Healthcare Improvement as well as the primary quality improvement method used by the authors. The Model for Improvement is a simple but robust model that can be applied to any QI project. The Model for Improvement provides a clearly defined framework for achieving change within an accelerated timeframe.

Changes are driven by 3 key questions:

1. What are we trying to accomplish?
2. How will we know that a change is an improvement?
3. What changes can we make that will result in improvement?

The Model for Improvement also dictates a very specific set of steps for improvement:

- establish a team
- create an aim statement
- determine a set of measures
- plan and test changes (PDSA cycles)
- spread and sustain changes

The Plan-Do-Study-Act (PDSA) cycle is a crucial element of the Model for Improvement. This design for quality process is attributed to Walter Shewhart. Initially called the Shewhart Cycle, it is now known as the PDSA cycle [9]. Small, rapid cycles of tests allow QI teams to explore ideas and identify successes and failures without investing significant time or resources. Using PDSA cycles, teams can quickly refine changes prior to implementing on a large scale. Measurement is a critical element in any improvement process. To appreciate the impact of change strategies, data must be displayed over time.

The Model for Improvement requires inclusion of stakeholders. Change cannot succeed without involving the people who will carry out the work, the front-line workers. Often management develops strategies to gain improvement and push it to the front line without first involving front-line members or testing ideas. Time, money, and morale are lost when the untested action plan subsequently fails. Employing the Model for Improvement framework to prompt change can promote efficiency and decrease cost.

The Model for Improvement is particularly well suited to the health care industry because of its emphasis on PDSA cycles [14]. The responsibility for patient welfare combined with an intense work pace and strict time constraints make small, rapid tests of change an ideal format for improvement. Healthcare institutions are complicated systems with complex approval channels; therefore, changes need to be thoroughly vetted before large scale implementation.

QI can be easily incorporated into any process or activity. At its most basic level, QI is a natural, logical process: identify an area for improvement, try out different solutions, and adopt the one that works best. The benefits of QI in healthcare are innumerable and range from increased safety and improved patient outcomes to decreased waste and enhanced cost savings. By current estimates, it takes 10 years for new treatments to reach patients; it is possible that QI can greatly reduce that gap. QI skills also benefit the patient through promotion ofenhanced teamwork and better outcomes.

QI has become a mainstay of U.S. business practice, but has not been adopted by the healthcare industry. One reason is the relative autonomy that the practice of medicine has traditionally employed. Healthcare organizations currently are fragmented and complex silos that would benefit from a standardized curriculum. To better foster the transformation of healthcare, QI education is a necessity for improvement in patient safety and quality of care.

There are many ways to format a QI curriculum. This chapter spotlights an innovative approach at the Center for Advancing Pediatric Excellence (CAPE)of the Department of Pediatrics at Carolinas Medical Center in Charlotte, North Carolina. A structured curriculum can make QI easily incorporated into daily work for residents and other staff by breaking the methodology into timely pieces. A stepped, hands-on curriculum further entrenches QI skills by establishing fundamentals and then building on each previous experience.

THE CAPE PROGRAM

CAPE was established in the Carolinas Medical Center (CMC) Department of Pediatrics in 2009 to educate residents in QI methodology, as well as practical application by participating in multidisciplinary QI teams including leadership roles.

When the ACGME began requiring residents to demonstrate QI knowledge, no specific guidelines or outcomes were mandated. In addition, there were few opportunities for residents to practice QI skills in the field. The CAPE curriculum was designed to provide a structure for a program that integrated QI skill development seamlessly into a larger resident curriculum.

A Duke Endowment grant intended to "strengthen an institution's QI capacity" provided initial funding for CAPE. The CAPE staff consists of a QI Coach, Data Analyst, and Program Coordinator.

The CAPE curriculum integrates education and improvement. Residents learn by active participation, and the program weaves multiple QI experiences into other residency activities over an extended period of time. By simultaneously learning QI fundamentals and practicing QI skills, residents gain the dexterity necessary to apply these skills to new and different challenges. This approach has the added benefit of producing institution-wide improvements and increased capacity by placing residents on interdisciplinary QI teams. A successful QI curriculum must go beyond unilateral knowledge transfer: action and discussion lie at the heart of QI. A successful curriculum must strategically apply adult learning theory concepts.

There are numerous theories of adult learning, often with competing view points of how knowledge is acquired in adulthood. In 1968, Knowles popularized the concept of andragogy and noted a distinct difference between how adults acquire knowledge compared to children. The learning concepts attributed to Knowles are self-direction, learning from previous experiences, readiness and willingness to learn, ease of application and motivation (internal). [15] More recently, Merriam points to transformational learning as the key to adult learning. [16] Transformational learning focuses on development of skills, experience and critical reflection. Critical reflection and development of deeper understanding is postulated to impact knowledge, skills and attitudes. Other key theories include relevance and applicability to practice as important factors in developing and retaining knowledge and having the ability to transfer learning to other situations. Similarly, Kolb and Fry's model of learning as a circular process consists of concrete experience, observation and reflection, the formation of abstract concepts and testing of concepts in new situations. [17] Although all of these models differ slightly in their approach, the similarities underscore that the adult learner has to be invested or engaged in the process of learning for the transfer of knowledge to be successful.

CURRICULUM

Participating in a QI project incorporates a focus on evidence-based practice as well as outcome measures. As described by Langley [13], education alone does not automatically translate into change. True improvement results from giving context to otherwise abstract concepts, and this connection is best made with real improvement projects. A common pitfall is to invest a disproportionate amount of effort in teaching without linking the knowledge to a tangible result. Research indicates that hands-on learning methods improve demonstrated skill levels, and the addition of coaching and review vastly elevate the learner's ability to apply skills to new situations. [13]

Residency programs, in an effort to address the ACGME requirements, have adopted many methods of providing QI education during residency. Numerous formats have been used to satisfy this requirement: didactic lectures, one month rotations, chart audits, and short QI projects. These formats do not incorporate QI into everyday practice and are less effective methods to embed QI methodology into daily practice. QI incorporation into daily practice requires hardwiring as a life-long skill.

The CAPE curriculum is a three-year longitudinal experience combining didactics, online tutorials, and independent readings with intensive guided experiences.

The CAPE curriculum and resident projects are developed with the Institute for Healthcare Improvement Triple Aim in mind – improve the health of children, enhance the patient experience, and control cost of care. [18] This curriculum utilizes a stepped approach, in the belief that building on previous experiences makes the skills more readily accessible and deeply ingrained. The ultimate goal is to integrate QI skills into "the way we do our work" rather than an additional responsibility.

A variety of education and training methods are used in the CAPE QI curriculum. Focus is on practice, participation on QI teams, and coaching and review which have been identified as highly effective methods of training. [13, 19]

Coaching promotes the implementation of new skills, as well as increased and correct usage. [19] One-on-one coaching is a cornerstone of the resident's experience for the first two years.

The QI Coach provides just-in-time teaching to suit each stage of a resident's QI development. A dedicated QI Coach provides the necessary support for various stages of resident QI projects. For example, one second-year resident's team may be struggling to establish the basic goal of a project while another second year's team is ready to analyze data and plan for sustainability.

The residents' first introduction to coaching is through the Personal Improvement Project. The Personal Improvement Project applies the Model for Improvement process to a personal, non-clinical improvement goal. For example, one resident used small, rapid tests to improve her consumption of fruits and vegetables (table 1). This portion of the curriculum is designed to introduce QI methodology and apply basic QI skills. With guidance from the QI Coach and Data Analyst, each resident develops an aim statement and data management plan, carries out tests of change, and continuously analyzes the results using run charts to determine which changes result in improvement. The first year residents present their projects at an internal educational conference.

After building on skills developed during the Personal Improvement Project, the remaining portion of the first year is devoted to a clinical Reflective Practice Project. The Reflective Practice Project is a chart audit exercise intended to help residents analyze gaps in their own practice in providing quality care (table 2). The QI Coach meets with residents during their ambulatory clinic rotations to instruct them about chart audits, help identify an area for improvement, and guide them through tests of change. In the future, the ability to get data directly from the electronic medical record in an aggregate fashion will potentially make chart auditing less necessary while the underlying concept remains. The Reflective Practice Project sets the stage for the resident to develop life-long skills of practice evaluation and critical reflection.

Table 1. Sample Personal Improvement Project

Aim Statement: Good nutrition can have positive impacts on many aspects of your life: physical health, energy level, mood, and more. Since starting residency, I have been going out to eat more often, eating a lot of processed food in the cafeterias, and not preparing many fresh meals at home. A balanced diet is an extremely important component of a balanced life. By November 30, 2011, I hope to improve my overall diet by eating more fresh foods, both at work and at home.

Goals:

-- I will prepare dinner at home at least 4 of 7 nights each week
-- I will eat at least 2 cups of fruit a day*

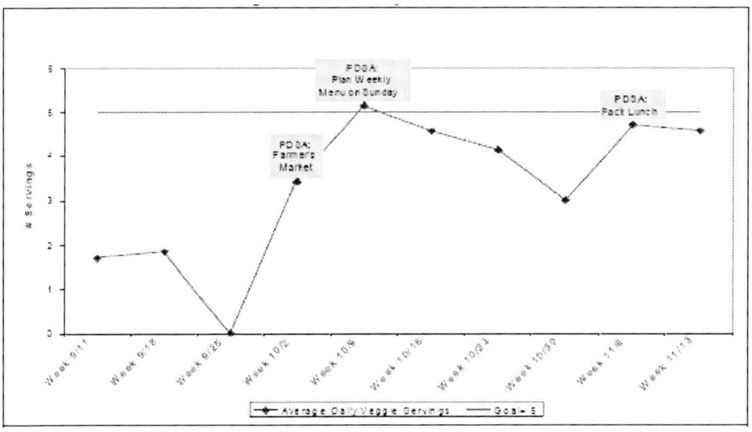

-- I will eat at least 2.5 cups of vegetables a day*
* *using CDC website for serving sizes*

Measure Set:

-- Number of home-cooked dinners each week
-- Servings of fruit each day
-- Servings of vegetables each day
-- Preparing dinner at home will take more time away from other activities (studying, exercising, social activities, etc.)

Sample PDSA cycles:

-- Incorporating fruit into each morning's breakfast
-- Packing lunch at home to bring to work
-- Making a dinner plan at the beginning of each week
-- Going to the farmers market for fresh fruits and veggies

Table 2. Sample Reflective Practice Projects

Topic	Target Population Age	Baseline Audit	Final Audit
Anticipatory Guidance – water safety	Newborn – 23 months	0%	78%
Age Appropriate Safety Education	Newborn – 4 years	50%	100%
Reach Out and Read – review and give book	6 months – 5 years	13%	100%

The Reflective Practice Project is not a complete QI project, as its data component is limited to only pre- and post-intervention on their continuity panel. The data burden is limited because the activity's main purposes are 1) to analyze gaps in care and 2) to hone the skills needed to test changes in small cycles. More intensive data education is included in the subsequent phase of the curriculum. As residents enter their second year, the QI skills are put into practice working on QI teams. Using institutional needs and resident preference, the QI Coach helps each resident make the shift into a team-based approach to QI. At this stage, residents also develop their knowledge of measures, outcomes, and sustainability. This portion of the curriculum represents the long term experiential learning of QI skills. Since residency has a complex rotational schedule with varying demands, the residents must find creative ways to contribute, such as developing an evidence-based protocol or algorithm to be tested as part of the QI project; likewise, residents may have to communicate with teammates through a virtual environment.

In keeping with institutional goals, resident projects are categorized into the areas of Patient Safety, Clinical Outcomes, and Clinical Efficiency (table 3). A sample project is summarized in table 4. This project is an implementation of the health literacy technique of Teach Back in a resident continuity clinic.

Table 3. Sample Resident Projects

Patient Safety	Clinical Outcomes	Clinical Efficiency
IV Antibiotic Family Education	ADHD	Team STEPPS
Hematology Oncology: Neutropenia	Asthma	Streamlining the Discharge Process
Hematology Oncology: Emergency Preparedness	Bright Futures	Resident Education Archive
SCAN (Child Abuse)	Obesity	Children's Hospital Inpatient Service Geography (Inpatient Placement Process)
Implementing Teach Back	Expedited Partner Treatment	Open Access and Office Efficiency
Transition from Teen to Adult Provider	Extremely Low Birth Weight (<500 gram)	Census Boards
Physical Abuse Inpatient Evaluation	Infant Mortality	

By their third year, residents are expected to fulfill a leadership role on an interdisciplinary inpatient or outpatient QI team. While working closely with the project's physician champion, residents draw heavily on QI Coach support. Third year residents may choose between stepping up on an existing project, directing a smaller spin-off project, or initiating a brand new project. Key roles include writing the aim statement, designing and executing PDSA cycles, establishing agendas and leading team meetings, delegating tasks to other team members,and helping create team member accountability. Every third year resident must present his or her project at an academic forum before graduation, either within the organization or nationally. Some current residents are planning to use their QI projects for publications.

Table 4. Case Study: Implementing Teach Back in a Pediatric Resident Clinic

Health literacy is the ability to read, understand and effectively use basic medical instructions and information. Low health literacy can affect anyone of any age, ethnicity, background or education level. Limited health literacy is a significant barrier to communicating with patients which affects access to health care services, understanding health information, and decreases patients' ability to make appropriate health care decisions. Limited health literacy results in negative health outcomes including: inability to understand medication directions, improper management of chronic disease, and poor compliance. All of these factors can result in unnecessary emergency room visits and increased hospitalizations. Residents represent the front line in medical care, and are in the ideal position to use an evidence-based health literacy tool such as Teach Back to improve their patients' health outcomes. Teach Back is a technique used to determine if information is understood by having the patient or parent explain in their own words. *Project Goals:* > 90% of well child visits the resident will utilize Teach Back > 90% of well child visits would be rated by staff and patient as very satisfied < 10% increase in cycle time for well child visits < 10% of patients would need to have Teach Back repeated *Intervention:* During well child care visits in the first year of life, a standardized teaching session was performed by a second year resident. Three age appropriate topics outlined in Bright Futures from American Academy of Pediatrics were discussed. The parent was encouraged to ask questions and then asked to Teach Back to the resident the three topics discussed. A nurse or an interpreter observed the Teach Back. If Teach Back was not successful, additional teaching was done and this time was added to the cycle time. Baseline cycle time data was collected by observing several second year residents during similar visits, utilizing standardized teaching but not requesting Teach Back. Staff and provider satisfaction data was collected by using a five point scale. Patient satisfaction was assessed using a scale to rate the visit and rate the interaction with the provider. Introduction of the Teach Back technique in resident continuity clinic achieved positive feedback from staff and providers. Patient satisfaction scores rated the intervention favorably. The cycle time of the office visit was not increased and actually decreased over time as the visit became more efficient. As the resident improved their technique of Teach Back, the knowledge transfer was more effective requiring less repeating of information. Utilization of the technique of Teach Back in the clinic setting improves communication and ensures that parents have the knowledge they need. Health literacy improvements can be made in a resident clinic without adding additional time to visits.

Providers have a greater sense of accomplishment and job satisfaction when the information they teach is truly learned.

Using the Train the Trainer method, the resident will train peers in the technique of Teach Back. The first control chart demonstrates cycle time among second year pediatric residents without any intervention. This process is stable, with the mean time of 25 minutes for a well child care visit and a median time of 23 minutes.

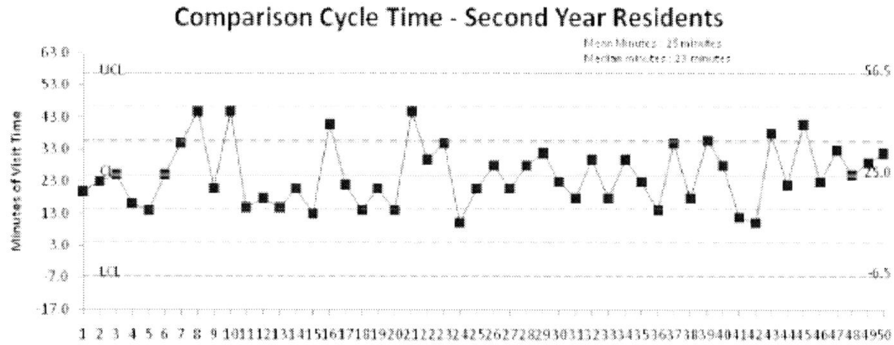

The second control chart demonstrates cycle time using the intervention of Teach Back during well child care visits. As demonstrated the control chart displays a special cause denoting a change in the process, in this case improvement. The mean visit time is 19.8 minutes and the median visit is 20 minutes.

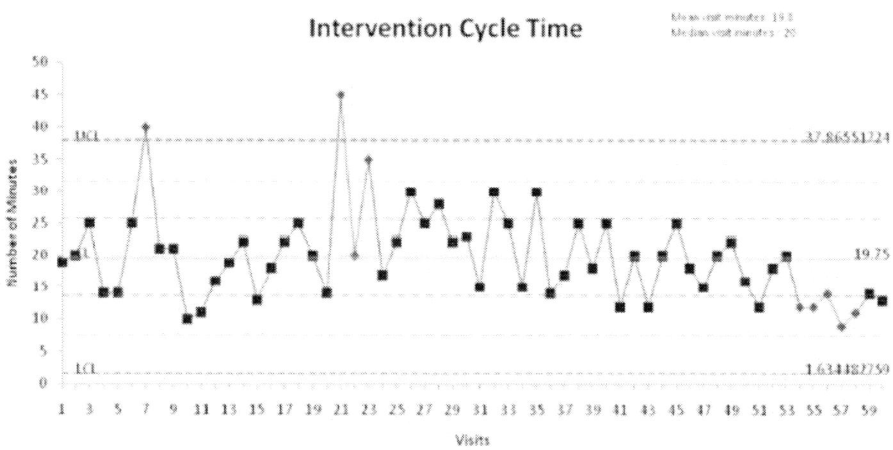

A primary principle of QI is sustainability. As residents prepare to graduate, they must either shift project responsibilities to a rising second or third year resident or establish a sustainability plan. This is an important but challenging final step in QI training; QI teams may lose the gains achieved by failing to hardwire changes. The written hand-off or sustainability plan is included in their final project report, and filed in their residency portfolio.

June 2012 marks an important milestone in CAPE's development, as the first group of residents to receive the full 3-year curriculum will graduate. These physicians will provide the most valuable feedback to date on the program's impact, both by reflecting on their complete experience and by future reporting on its usefulness in the field. The ultimate affirmation of the curriculum may be whether CAPE-trained pediatricians continue to embed QI skills and practice improvement throughout their career.

Resident self reports of QI knowledge and skill have increased with each year of the CAPE curriculum. A survey is completed by the residents at the beginning and end of each program year. The resident identifies the ability to use QI methods and tools and responses based on a Likert scale ranging from not confident to extremely confident. Overall, residents report an increase in confidence in application of QI knowledge and skill.

By introducing QI through the Personal Improvement Project, learners are immediately immersed in QI science, and gain dexterity with the skills as abstract concepts rapidly transform into concrete results with supporting data. This hands-on approach also promotes future use of the skill set by demonstrating its intuitive nature.

Intensive individualsupport also shifts learning from a passive to an active format. One-on-one coaching facilitates a dynamic, back-and-forth discussion that is radically different from the more traditional lecture format. The QI Coach tailors teaching to specific situations; the result is that learners immediately and actively apply methodology to their work. Furthermore, because the QI Coach tracks resident advancement through the curriculum, activity-based milestones are more uniformly met.

CAPE curriculum's stepped approach also reinforces an action-based approach to learning. By building on each previous activity, the program more fully integrates the skill set into physicians' daily work. As learners use the methodology to resolve more and more challenges, they are inspired to continue drawing on this skill set. The full spectrum of the curriculum – beginning with the Personal Improvement Project and ending with a leadership role – ensures practitioners have mastered each step before advancing to the next.

CAPE leaders regularly apply QI principles to the curriculum, and identified opportunities for improvement in the use of data. Knowledge gaps in the areas of patient safety – especially human factor engineering and reliability – are being added to the curriculum.

While residents' data-related skills have improved, there is still great opportunity for advancement. In the past, many teams did not have sufficient data to drive change. Continuous coaching is necessary to prompt teams to assess their data on an ongoing basis with a focus on data-driven improvement. As residents become more proficient with data methodology, more sophisticated subject matter will be incorporated with more efficient methods of data collection.

BUILDING ORGANIZATIONALCAPACITY: QI EDUCATION BEYOND THE RESIDENCY

One of QI's major goals is to break down silos and divisions that hamper rapid improvement. Consequently, QI education needs to be fostered institution-wide. Department and hospital leadership support QI, and because successful QI cannot take place in a vacuum, part of CAPE's mandate include educating a wide range of other hospital and clinic staff. This allows residents and other providers (e.g. physicians, nurses, registration staff, social workers, etc.) to implement QI projects from a common foundation. System-wide education ensures a seamless collaboration between residents and teams. CAPE accomplishes this system-wide education by sharing fundamental pieces of the curriculum in a condensed format. Staff learning opportunities include participating in a monthly 2-hour QI Orientation taught by CAPE staff and attending or presenting at QI Forums held each April, August, and December. The QI Orientation introduces QI methodology and gives audience members hands-on practice identifying improvement opportunities and planning changes to test. The QI Forum is a multidisciplinary system-wide conference for the exchange of current QI projects within the institution. It allows residents and staff to present their QI projects and engage in open discussion with the audience. This 2-hour event also features QI didactics by CAPE staff. Together these two educational series further standardize QI education across the facility.

QI coaching is also a valuable educational resource for the entire facility. Coaching consultations are provided by CMC's Quality Department and the CAPE QI Coach. The QI Coach ensures residents have a positive, productive experience, and also exposes the entire team to real-time application of QI methodology and implementation of QI tools.

Shared learning is an important QI tool, with the capacity to vastly expedite QI spread. To this end, CAPE orchestrates Institute for Healthcare Improvement-style collaboratives that bring multiple facility teams together to work on complementary changes. This process weaves QI education with subject-specific information such as health literacy and office efficiency, and helps standardize QI knowledge across the facility. The efforts of the CAPE QI initiative strengthen the improvement capability of the organization thus strengthening the institution and the care provided to patients.

Standardized education and training can also be accomplished through faculty development and continuing medical education (CME) for physicians, and through continuing education credits (CEUs) for other health care disciplines. ACCME requirements to include QI in continuing education can be satisfied in a variety of ways:

1) teaching project-based QI courses
2) incorporating QI methodology into medical content courses
3) conducting learning collaboratives which combine medical content and QI education in a project framework

These learning opportunities can be conducted in face-to-face environments or through web-based courses. CAPE directors and staff have developed curriculums for each of these scenarios, and participate as faculty, directors, or coordinators.

Institutional and administrative leaders are crucial to the success of any QI endeavor, particularly adoption of a QI curriculum. As a general rule, leader support greatly enhances a QI project's progress: increases participants' accountability, alleviates barriers, promotes spread and hardwiring, and provides needed resources. Because a QI curriculum has the potential to impact the entire institution, support from administration is essential. The agreement and collaboration between the hospital president, chief medical officer, residency director, and assistant vice presidents of patient care services and outpatient services, as well as CAPE's director and co-director was essential in implementation and sustainability. These leaders pledged valuable resources during the program's inception, facilitate team progress, and continue to work together to integrate resident QI programming into the broader staff experience. These individuals are active members of the CAPE steering committee, and work with CAPE staff, faculty, and data specialists to ensure teams and projects achieve their goals.

Conclusion

Spread is an important step in the QI process, and one that encompasses the most important principles of QI. Sharing a team's experience expedites improvement and maximizes the impact of their work. It prevents other teams from having to re-invent the wheel, and ensures that the team's effort and investment go farther. Standardization is a hallmark of successful QI endeavors. Ensuring that everyone follows the same process and shares the same knowledge base allows team success. To this end, CAPE has shared the curriculum with other residency programs at CMC, and is disseminating curriculum components to other institutions.

While the authors firmly believe the CAPE program is most effective in its complete format, they recognize it may not be possible for every institution to implement the entire curriculum. However, it is possible to separate and adapt various pieces to fit the needs of any institution. The curriculum is designed as a change package of 6 primary elements. These 6 are:

- Didactics
- Independent learning
- Individualized coaching
- PersonalImprovement Project
- Reflective Practice Project
- Membership on QI team

For example one institution could pair independent learning with the Personal Improvement Project, while another chooses to combine didactics with a Reflective Practice Projectand membership on a QI team. Three secondary elements remain that are vital to fulfillment of a comprehensive longitudinal curriculum: leadership of a QI team, scholarly presentation of QI project, and development of a QI sustainability plan. These items may be difficult to undertake without extensive infrastructure and support.

It is possible to implement some aspects of the CAPE program on a limited budget. For example, the self-directed learning can be obtained free of cost. In addition to a wide variety of independent reading available, as of this writing the Institute for Healthcare Improvement (IHI) offers online tutorials at no charge to students, medical residents, and university faculty; other health professionals can access the courses for a modest cost. Small grants can be pursued to fund an educational QI agenda or be integrated into an existing resident curriculum. Institutions interested in implementing QI education can hire a single coach or coordinator to work with residents, without employing a full-scale center with directors, data support, and program manager. Even without a dedicated staff position, the residency program director can include self-directed learning requirements in the graduating residents' portfolios.

Learning by doing is the foundation of the CAPE program and its most important teaching technique. Almost all hospitals and community organizations have Quality or Patient Safety initiatives which residents can join. By actively participating on a QI team, residents learn practical application of the institution's preferred methodology. At the next level of investment, QI students can attend one of the IHI's many conference offerings. These learning opportunities include sessions ranging from novice to master experience levels.

The CAPE curriculum, with its combination of self-directed learning and structured quality improvement practice, promotes the skills required for life-long learning. This quality improvement curriculum adapts known QI methodology and practice to the local context or the home organization's established QI program.

QI education that is integrated into a medical curriculum on both the graduate and undergraduate level has the potential to transform the delivery of medical care. This transformation can improve outcomes, eliminate waste, improve efficiency, foster teamwork and increase patient safety. The necessary skills can be incorporated into medical curriculums assuring that medical providers of the future deliver patient-centered quality healthcare. Providers currently in practice who have not received training in QI will require education as the entire healthcare delivery system is being revamped to reward desirable outcomes.

REFERENCES

[1] A. Flexner, *Medical Education in the United* , Bulletin No. 4, The Carnegie Foundation for the Advancement of Teaching, New York City(1910).

[2] A. H. Beck, "The Flexner Report and the Standardization of American Medical Education", *JAMA: the Journal of the American Medical Association*291 (17): 2139–2140 (2004).

[3] Accreditation Council for Graduate Medical Education (ACGME), "ACGME Approved Standards: Common Program Requirements." Accessed March 27, 2012. http://acgme-2010standards.org/pdf/ Common_Program_Requirements_07012011.pdf.

[4] Institute of Medicine U.S. Committee on Quality of Health Care in America, *Crossing the Quality Chasm: A new health system for the 21st century*, National Academy Press, Washington, DC (2001).

[5] Accreditation Council for Continuing Medical Education (ACCME),*The Accreditation Council for Continuing Medical Education at Work: Accreditation, Recognition, Education, Operations, and Governance* (2010).

[6] M. Cooke, D. M. Irby, and B. C. O'Brien, *Educating Physicians: A Call for Reform of Medical School and Residency*, Jossey-Bass, San Francisco (2010).

[7] J. Juran, *Quality Control Handbook*, McGraw-Hill, New York (1951).

[8] W. E. Deming, *Out of the Crisis*, MIT Press (1986).

[9] W. A.Shewhart,*The economic control of quality of manufactured product* (1931). Reprinted by American Society for Quality Control, Milwaukee (1980).

[10] J. F. Krafcik, "Triumph of the lean production system",*Sloan Management Review*30 (1): 41–52(1988).

[11] D. H. Stamatis, *Six Sigma Fundamentals: A Complete Guide to the System, Methods, and Tools*, Productivity Press, New York(2004).

[12] K. Walshe, G. Harvey, P. Jas,*Connecting Knowledge and Performance in Public Services: From Knowing to Doing*, Cambridge University Press(2010).

[13] G. J. Langley, R. D. Moen, K. M. Nolan, T. W. Nolan, C. L. Norman, L. P. Provost,*The Improvement Guide: A practical approach to enhancing organizational performance*, 2nd Edition,Jossey-Bass,San Francisco (2009).

[14] C.D. Courtlandt, L. Noonan, L. G. Feld, "Model for Improvement – Part 1: A Framework for Health Care Quality," *PediatrClin N Am* 56: 757-778 (2009).

[15] M. S. Knowles, *The Modern Practice of Adult Education from Pedagogy to Andragogy*, 2nd Edition, New York Cambridge Books (1980).
[16] S. B. Merriam and R. S. Caffarella,*Learning in adulthood: A comprehensive guide*, 2ndEdition,Jossey-Bass,San Francisco(1999).
[17] D. A. Kolb and R. Fry,"Toward an applied theory of experiential learning", in C. Cooper(ed), *Theories of Group Process*, John Wiley, London (1975).
[18] Institute for Healthcare Improvement, "The Triple Aim", *Healthcare Executive* 24: 64-66 (2009).
[19] B. Joyce and B. Showers, *Student Achievement through Staff Development*,3rd Edition, Association for Supervision and Curriculum Development, Alexandria, VA (2002).

Section Three: Patient Safety

In: Quality Improvement
Editors: K. W. Lobdell and S. C. Stamou
ISBN: 978-1-62417-390-5

Chapter 4

PATIENT SAFETY: AN OVERVIEW

***Juan A. Sanchez*[1] *and Kevin W. Lobdell*[2]**
[1]Department of Surgery, Saint Mary's Hospital,
University of Connecticut Health Center, Farmington, CT, US
[2]Cardiothoracic Surgery, Sanger Heart and Vascular Institute,
Carolinas HealthCare System, University of North Carolina
School of Medicine, Charlotte, NC, US

ABSTRACT

The increasing recognition that, despite spectacular progress in treating disease and improving health, health care can be unsafe for patients has triggered a considerable reassessment of contemporary medical practice in the context of a complex and opaque system. The science of human error and theoretical concepts from other safety-critical industries are increasingly relevant to the emerging interprofessional discipline of Patient Safety. Many challenges remain ahead to achieve safety and high-reliability from our health care delivery system.

INTRODUCTION

In any patient-centered healthcare delivery system, safety is the foundation for quality. Unsafe systems, unmitigated hazards, near-misses, and other safety-related issues are the "low hanging fruit" of all quality improvement efforts. In general, when a patient interacts with a healthcare institution, it is an expected societal norm that the provider is competent and capable of choosing and executing contextually appropriate methods of care for that individual. Deviations from this expectation, whether resulting in harm to the patient or not, violate the traditional trust awarded to institutions of healing by society at large. While definitions of medical error and adverse events are subject to vigorous debate, there is ample evidence that the healthcare environment is dangerous and can unintentionally harm patients.

Patient Safety is emerging as an interprofessional, multidisciplinary specialty with a theoretical framework drawing from many other safety-critical industries. This new healthcare discipline emphasizes the reporting, analysis of events and near misses, "hardwiring" optimal healthcare practices in order to eliminate adverse events. The Patient Safety movement has emerged as a coalition of a variety of stakeholders which include providers, patients, financing bodies, and the general public. This discipline is increasingly supported by a growing body of literature from within the healthcare 'space' as well as by the increasing interest and involvement of safety experts from other fields eager to apply lessons learned to the complex and seemingly intractable problem of patient safety.

Childbed Fever and the Epidemiologic Approach to Patient Safety

1840's Vienna saw an alarming rate of "childbed" (puerperal) fever with considerable mortality for both mother and child following delivery. While many elaborate theories regarding the nature of this disease were put forth at the time, it became apparent to German-Hungarian physician, Ignaz Semmelweis that the prevalence of this condition varied between different obstetrical clinics. Analyzing data from clinic records at the Vienna General Hospital, Semmelweis identified a difference in rates of puerperal fever between two separate maternity clinics [1, 2]. He correlated a rise in the rate of this condition at the clinic attended by physicians with the institution of post-mortem examinations whereas the other the maternity clinic exclusively staffed by midwives did not experience an increase in childbed fever (Figure 1). Furthermore, he demonstrated that, by instituting hand washing with chloride of lime in 1847, the rate of this dreaded condition decreased to levels found at the midwife-staffed clinic.

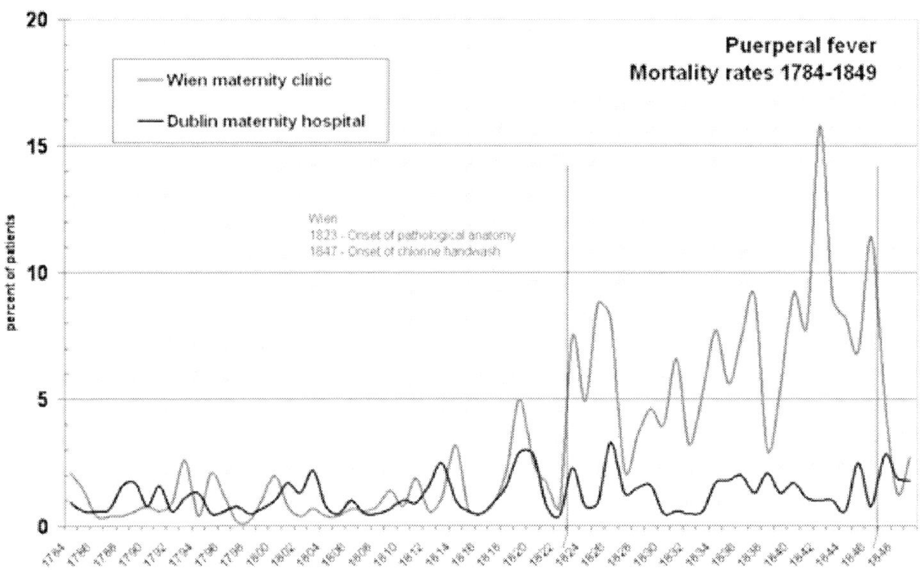

Figure 1. Mortality rates for childbed (Puerperal) fever at separate maternity wards [35].

In the 19th century, the idea that physicians themselves could transfer pathogens from the autopsy room to maternity patients resulting in their death was shocking. Nevertheless, these events laid the groundwork for hospital epidemiology and efforts to control healthcare associated infections.

THE SCOPE AND PREVALENCE OF HEALTHCARE HARM

The Institute of Medicine's report "To Err is Human," in 1999 which estimated that medical errors result in about between 44,000 and 98,000 preventable deaths and 1,000,000 excess injuries each year in U.S. hospitals making it the tenth leading cause of death has become a clarion call alerting healthcare organizations, regulators, and the public to the alarming incidence of medical errors [3]. The report highlighted the complexity and system design issues in contemporary health care delivery and provided a framework for rebuilding the system for safety. Previously, several studies had pointed out the existence of inconsistent medical practice resulting in patient harm suggesting that the problem was underappreciated and widespread. For example, a Harvard Medical study in 1991 concluded that patients incurred a substantial amount of injury during medical treatment as a result of substandard care [4].

In the United States, approximately 10% of acute hospital admissions result in an adverse event [5]. It has been estimated that the IOM report considerably underestimates the problem. For example, a study published in 2000 suggests that as many as 225,000 people die from iatrogenic causes, making it the third leading cause of death [6].

A report from the Inspector General of the U.S. Department of Health and Human Services on a nationally representative random sample of 780 Medicare beneficiaries discharged in October, 2008, estimated that 27% experienced either temporary or permanent harm or death during their hospital stays [7]. Physician reviewers determined that, at least, 44 % of these events were clearly or likely preventable. Furthermore, hospital care associated with harm events cost the Medicare Program an estimated $324 million for one month alone. A study in the Journal of the American Medical Association involving hospitals under the Department of Veterans Affairs estimated that one patient died for lack of optimal care for roughly every 10,000 patients admitted [8]. Other studies have shown that up to 30 % of patients receive care that is contraindicated [9]. While the methodological approaches can be argued, the literature points to a widespread problem, at least for hospitalized patients. Data to determine the prevalence of medical harm in the outpatient setting, however, remains sorely lacking.

Studies suggest that the problem of patient safety is not limited to the U.S. Other countries, with fundamentally different systems of healthcare delivery and financing are not immune. In Canada, for example, 7.5 % of hospital admissions resulted in an adverse event according to one study [10, 11]. Nearly a quarter of Canadians reported they or a family member had experienced a preventable adverse event due to medical care with half of the events resulting in serious consequences. A RAND Corporation study has concluded that, in the United Kingdom, 10.3 % of acute hospital admissions resulted in adverse event deaths resulted from adverse care events, 36 from adverse drug events [12]. In 2000, the Department of Health Expert Group estimated that over 850,000 incidents of harm in hospitalized patients occurred in the National Health Service (NHS) each year and that forty incidents contribute to deaths at each NHS hospital each year [13]. Elsewhere in Europe, the rate of adverse events leading to death in hospitalized patients ranks ahead of air pollution, substance abuse, and trauma [12, 14]. An Australian study revealed 18,000 annual deaths from medical errors [15]. In New Zealand, 12.3 % of acute hospital admissions result in the incidence of an adverse event [16]. The World Health Organization estimates that one in ten persons receiving health care will suffer preventable harm [17].

Table 1. Common Adverse Events in Hospitalized Patients

Adverse Events	Examples
Hospital –Acquired Infections (HAI)	Ventilator-Associated Pneumonia (VAP) Central Line-Associated Bloodstream Infection (*CLABSI*)
Adverse Drug Reactions	Penicillin administration despite known allergy
Identification Errors	Wrong blood type transfusion Wrong side, wrong site, wrong patient
Injury or Failure to Prevent Injury	Patient Falls and Restraint-Related Injuries Unnecessary radiation exposure Patient Suicide Operating room burns from fires, cautery pads, chemicals
Design-related/Device Related Injury	Implantable defibrillator misfires
Memory Lapses	Retained Foreign Objects
Communication Failures	Illegible Doctor's orders Improper sign-out at shift change

While the response to this call to action by healthcare providers, governmental agencies, and other stakeholders has been vigorous, little evidence exists that progress has been made towards reducing errors and creating a safe environment for patients [18]. Moreover, patient harm is woefully underreported even internally within the institution [19]. In an in-depth review of 293 adverse events, 40 were reported to hospital administration and, of those, only 28 were investigated by the hospitals. Only five events led to changes in policies or practices. This absence of internal transparency prevents institutions from tracking errors and adverse events, analyzing their causes, ultimately improving care.

A number of Federal regulatory efforts in the U.S. and elsewhere have created opportunities for improvement through policy approaches which include non-payment for "never events" for government-sponsored health plans.

In 2005, The Patient Safety and Quality Improvement Act created whistleblower protection for reporting errors and implemented a voluntary reporting system [20]. As of 2012, only 27 states in the U.S. have laws requiring hospitals to publicly report hospital-acquired infections, from 6 in 2005 [21].

The health-services research community has, furthermore, expansively studied many of the cognitive, social, and operational elements which contribute to adverse events and have created interventions to mitigate errors and reduce these events using myriad approaches ranging from memory aides such as checklists to measuring an organization's culture often borrowing ideas, techniques, and tools from other safety-critical industries along the way. A number of tools have included safety climate assessment, effective teamwork training, examining provider fatigue, and reassessing the overall environment through a human factors lens. While there is, currently, no mandatory national reporting system for adverse events in the U.S., many "blameless" mechanisms have been developed by different institutions and systems for reporting harm events, unsafe conditions, and "close calls" with variable adoption. Payment systems, via either incentives or penalties for certain types of adverse events have recently been put in place. Whether these approaches lead to reduced medical errors and improved patient safety remains to be seen. [22]

DEFINING ERROR

In order to improve the quality of care and to better determine the fundamental sources of patient harm, a broad view of adverse events in the healthcare environment has been widely adopted. For example, the Institute for Healthcare Improvement (IHI) defines medical harm as the "unintended physical injury resulting from or contributed to by medical care (including the absence of indicated medical treatment), that requires additional monitoring, treatment or hospitalization, or that results in death. Such injury is considered harm whether or not it is considered preventable, whether or not it resulted from a medical error, and whether or not it occurred within a hospital" [23]. This expanded definition, implying neither intent nor negligence, reflects the potential for harm an increasingly complex and potentially dangerous system.

While frank negligence constitutes only a small fraction of adverse outcomes (about 1% according to the Harvard Medical Practice Study), lapses and mistakes are actually very common in healthcare. Additionally, it is increasingly evident that medical treatments offered patients are subject influence by a variety of non-patient related factors which can result in suboptimal care. Lack of available evidence, in the past, has allowed wide variations in medical treatments for a given condition as well as creating significant geographic differences and disparities in the type of treatment a patient is likely to receive [24]. Studies suggest that adults receive only 55% of the care recommended for a particular condition, while others suggest that certain types of treatments are over utilized and not indicated in as many as 30% of those receiving it [25, 26].

IATROGENESIS VS. COMEOGENESIS

The Hippocratic admonition against harming the sick while attempting to heal is rooted in the idea of a fiduciary relationship between patient and healer. This concept of non-maleficence remains a core value of modern bioethics. Theories abound regarding the historical influences which have impacted the evolution of this relationship over centuries. Some, for example, point out the possible influences of paternalism and pecuniary considerations as potential sources of the lack of improvement in the level of medical harm. In addition, the increasing pace of scientific and technological progress, with increasingly more potent treatments, has amplified the consequences of error in healthcare without fundamentally redesigning the system in which that care is delivered to account for the added risk [27]. It is becoming clear that the increasing level of complexity of the system, with the attendant potential for propagating and amplifying errors down a sequence of tightly coupled processes, along with diffuse accountability, and external pressures to function at the margins of capacity calls for a radical reevaluation of the system's overall design.

In contradistinction to the term "iatrogenesis" in which harm is caused as a result of an individual physician (Iatros = Greek for physician), the term "comeogenesis" bring to bear the broad notion that disease and its treatment bring negative effects to the patient's sense of well-being. As such, these terms are congruent with ideas emerging from error science in which "sharp-end" (direct) errors may be rooted in and be manifestations of system characteristics or the "blunt end", which create opportunities for mistakes, lapses, and unintended events.

Adverse outcomes due to the nature of the disease have often been difficult to differentiate from preventable harm as a result of unintended consequences of care. Interventions such as invasive procedures or pharmacotherapy with definable rates of complications are often indistinguishable from substandard medical care. Moreover, the difference between expected and unexpected complications is less obvious given the vagaries of physiologic responses to treatment. Increasingly, evidence-based medicine and treatment paradigms such as care pathways are important tools in standardizing processes of care. In addition, genomic technologies which identify those at risk for particular drug interactions or to select optimal care for individuals are becoming increasingly relevant to the nature of patient safety and medical harm.

THE SCIENCE OF HUMAN ERROR

Accident causation investigation has yielded valuable insight into factors contributing to error. Many theories have emerged from a variety of safety-critical industries regarding the nature of accidents and hazards. Complex socio-technical systems such as aviation and engineering understand the inevitability of error in human systems. A variety of conceptual frameworks have attempted to understand human error and typically describe such errors in the context of system design and the cumulative effects of various, seemingly small, failures percolating through gaps in the system's defenses ultimately resulting in an accident. British psychologist James T. Reason has theorized that most accidents are caused by at least one of four types of failure: organizational influences, unsafe supervision, preconditions for unsafe acts, and the unsafe acts themselves [28]. His Swiss Cheese Model of accident causation (Figure 2) imagines a system with various layers of defenses as slices of cheese. When the holes align, those ever-present conditions which trigger accidents are allowed through. The holes in the slices represent individual weaknesses in parts of the system dynamically changing in size and position.

In Reason's Model, errors are composed of either active failures, unsafe acts directly linked to harm, or latent failures which represent those conditions and system design elements which contribute or fail to prevent error [29].

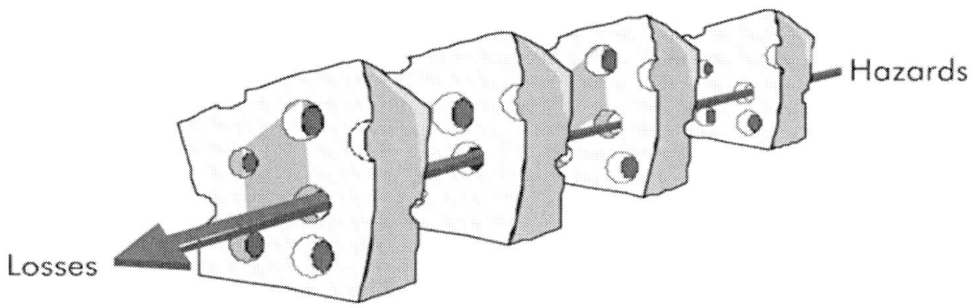

Figure 2. The Swiss Cheese Model. Each slice of cheese represents an organization's protective barriers to hazards. The barriers and their gaps (holes) are constantly changing in size and location (after Reason) [28].

The Swiss Cheese Model, among others, has been helpful in understanding errors and failures in the healthcare environment. It is complemented by a number of ideas and innovations to enhance performance and safety from the field of engineering and related disciplines such as Human Factors and Ergonomics, as well as techniques from group oriented industries such as Crew Resource Management.

Causes of Error in Healthcare

Unfortunately, a prevalent misconception regarding the causes of medical errors in that they are ultimately a result of careless or incompetent health care providers or “bad apples”. The increasing volume and complexity of healthcare services, along with increasing time pressure on providers and institutions under considerable fiscal constraints, all conspire to create abundant opportunities for accidents and errors. In addition, the fragmented access to patient data, inconsistent communication patterns, and movement of patients and providers in and out of organizations and health systems present formidable barriers to effective and reliable processes of care [30].

Systemic issues contributing to errors, decreased performance, and harm abound. The healthcare environment is target-rich for efforts to mitigate and eliminate hazards.

One of the most prevalent and obvious latent conditions reflect fragmented models of care and poor coordination resulting in an increased number of handoffs among the various components of the system across the entire spectrum of the patient’s disease. The rapid shift in demographics resulting from increased longevity as well as the increasing abundance of patients with chronic illnesses, create more exposure to the healthcare system and, of course, more opportunities for error. Furthermore, inadequate systems and incentives to share information regarding errors impede the ability to analyze and learn from causative factors.

Human Factors and Ergonomics

The multidisciplinary field of Human Factors and Ergonomics attempts to understand interactions among humans and other elements of a system, particularly in the context of complex, powerful technology. It applies theories and engineering principles to data obtained from various systems in order to design and optimize system performance and overall safety. It takes account of the user's capabilities and limitations in seeking to ensure that tasks, functions, relevant information, and the environment suit each user. The radically different lens through which Human Factors Engineers looks at healthcare often results in the identification of a variety of conditions and design features which can cause system failure. For example, the design of containers for powerful drugs so that they are not misidentified and the design of canisters and nozzles so that oxygen tubes cannot be confused with CO_2 tubes are examples of the value these engineering concepts bring to the system. Similar perspectives in workflow design and operations management can “hardwire” forcing functions to prevent errors and injury.

Communication Failures

Poor or ineffective communication is a major risk factor to patient safety. According to The Joint Commission, communication is the most common root cause of sentinel events in all categories constituting more than 70% of events reported of which approximately 75% are associated with death [31]. There are many reasons for communication failures including the fast pace of the work flow, the stressful environment of caring for ill patients, as well as cultural factors such as a historical climate of autonomy and hierarchy that often stifles the ability for individuals to speak up. Other sources of communication failures include the central role of paper-based processes in which legibility is inconsistent the increasing need to simultaneously inform multiple in a decentralized, highly compartmentalized and complex healthcare organization.

Moreover, the increasing reliance on team-based functions to deliver care has outstripped historical rules for dyadic communication exchanges particularly at crucial points in time such as patient handoffs or communication of critical lab values.

Structured forms of communication explicitly reduce ambiguity and enhance clarity. Such strategies facilitate effective information exchange by forcing the standardized and timely transfer of relevant and actionable data in a reliable way. It mandates, for example, that providers initiate a message during vulnerable, safety-critical periods in a properly coded format for optimal understanding. The consumer of the information is then required to acknowledge receipt of the information and reinterpret to data to ensure proper decoding.

In this fashion structured communication in the healthcare environment can improve the coordination of care delivery consistently. Requiring read-backs, use of Situation-Background-Assessment-Recommendation (SBAR) at handoffs as well as briefings, and debriefings and memory aids such as checklists are increasingly being implemented in the healthcare setting with promising results.

Examples of communication failures abound. In one study, trained observers recorded observations in the Operating Room during 48 surgical procedures involving 421 communication events. Communication failures occurred in approximately 30% of team exchanges and a third of these resulted in effects which jeopardized patient safety by increasing cognitive load, delays, interruptions, resource waste, and increasing the tension in the OR [32]. Other types of communication failures, however, involve the inability to transmit or receive information due to cognitive workload, implicit assumptions, authority gradients, lack of role clarity, and diffusion of responsibility. These, more intractable, problems are related to organizational cultures, workflow design, and current medical training paradigms.

Other Types of Errors

Wide variations exist in the experience and training of healthcare providers. Individual practitioner competency is often not rigorously evaluated either at the time of new hire or on an ongoing basis. Teaching hospitals are particularly exposed to varying levels of clinical proficiency, knowledge, and skill particularly early in the academic year when the so-called "July Effect" arguably may result in an increase in medication errors [33]. The incidence of misdiagnosis and under-diagnosis as well as overtreatment remains objects of considerable speculation as is the rate of unnecessary procedures.

Moreover, organizational cultures differ in the ability to identify and learn from error or near misses [34, 35]. High performing hospitals and healthcare systems have been able to incorporate learning from mistakes and failures. In fact, such learning organizations learn not only from each adverse event when it occurs but look at errors and procedural violations as tremendous opportunities for learning. High-reliability healthcare organizations, like their brethren in other industries are preoccupied with failure.

CONCLUSION

This Chapter has provided an overview of fundamental concepts related to patient safety. Specific activities and interventions designed to reduce adverse events in the healthcare environment is beyond the intended scope of the chapter.

However, the discipline of patient safety practice is at its infancy and progress is anticipated to escalate. No doubt, advancements in social and engineering sciences coupled with technological progress will allow healthcare organizations of the future to embed safety into core operations in order to reduce and, perhaps, eliminate events which produce harm to patients during and following exposure to the healthcare delivery system.

REFERENCES

[1] Semmelweis IP. *The cause, concept and prophylaxis of childbed fever* 1861.

[2] Hanninen, OM, Farago, E. Monos. Ignaz Semmelweis: the prophet of bacteriology. *Infect. Control*, 1983, vol. 4(5), pp.367-370.

[3] Kohn L, Corrigan J, Donaldson M. *To Err. Is Human: Building a Safer Health System.* Washington, D.C.: National Academies Press, 1999.

[4] Brennan TA, Leape LL, Laird NM, et al. Incidence of adverse events and negligence in hospitalized patients. Results of the Harvard Medical Practice Study I. *N. Engl. J. Med.* 1991;324:370-6.

[5] Leape LL. Errors in Medicine. *Clin. Chim. Acta.* 2009;404(1): 2–5.

[6] Starfield B. Is US Health Really the Best in the World? *JAMA.* 2000; 284(4):483–5.

[7] Levinson DR. *Adverse events in hospitals: national incidence among Medicare beneficiaries.* Department of Health and Human Services Office of Inspector General, November 2010 (OEI-06-09-00090).

[8] Hayward RA, Hofer TP. Estimating hospital deaths due to medical errors: preventability is in the eye of the reviewer. *JAMA.* 2001; 286(4): 415–20.

[9] Schuster MA, McGlynn EA, Brook RH. How good is the quality of health care in the United States? *Milbank Q.* 1998; 76(4):517–63.

[10] MacDermaid LJ (2005), *First, Do No Harm: Medical Error in Canada.*

[11] Baker GR, Norton PG, Flintoft V, et al. The Canadian Adverse Events Study: the incidence of adverse events among hospital patients in Canada. *CMAJ.* 2004;170(11):1678–85.

[12] Conklin A, Vilamovska A, de Vries H, Hatziandreu E. *Improving Patient Safety in the EU: Assessing the expected effects of three policy areas for future action.* 2008 RAND Corporation.

[13] Department of Health Expert Group (2000). *An organisation with a memory.* Department of Health, United Kingdom. Retrieved 2006-07-01.

[14] Schiøler T, Lipczak H, Pedersen BL, et al. Incidence of adverse events in hospitals. A retrospective study of medical records (Article in Danish). *Ugeskr. Laeg.* 2001;163(39):5370–78.

[15] Wilson RM, Runciman WB, Gibberd RW, et al. The Quality in Australian Health Care Study. *Med. J. Aust.* 1995;163(9):458–71.
[16] Adverse Events in New Zealand Public Hospitals: *Principal Findings from a National Survey"*. New Zealand Ministry of Health. December 2001.
[17] World Health Organization:10 facts on patient safety. Accessed 2008-05-19.
[18] Brady J, Ho K, Clancy CM. The quality and disparities reports: why is progress so slow? *Am. J. Med. Qual.* 2008 Sep-Oct;23(5):396-8.
[19] Levinson DR. *Hospital Incident Reporting Systems Do Not Capture Most Patient Harm.* Department of Health and Human Services Office of Inspector General, January 2012 (OEI-06-09-00091).
[20] Starfield B, Shi L, Macinko J. Physicians and quality: answering the wrong question. *Health Aff.* (Millwood). 2009; 28(2):596–7.
[21] Spencer A, Sward D, Ward J. *Lessons From the Pioneers: Reporting Healthcare-Associated Infections.* Washington, D.C.: National Conference of State Legislators;2010.
[22] Leape LL, Berwick DM. Five years after to err is human: what have we learned? *JAMA.* 2005;293(19):2384–90.
[23] www.IHI.org.
[24] Wennberg JE, Cooper MM, eds. The quality of medical care in the United States: A report on the Medicare program. In: *The Dartmouth atlas of health care 1999.* American Health Association, Chicago, IL.
[25] McGlynn EA, Asch SM, Adams J, et al. The quality of health care delivered to adults in the United States. *N. Engl. J. Med.* 2003; 348(26): 2635-45.
[26] Fisher ES. Medical care: Is more always better? *N. Engl. J. Med.* 2003; 349(17): 1665–67.
[27] Sharpe and Faden Medical Harm.
[28] Reason, James (1990-10-26). *Human Error.* Cambridge University Press.
[29] Wiegmann DA, Shappell SA. A Human Error Approach to Aviation Accident Analysis: *The Human Factors Analysis and Classification System.* Ashgate Publishing, Ltd. 2003 pp. 48–49.
[30] Conklin A, Vilamovska A, de Vries H, et al. Improving Patient Safety in the EU Assessing the expected effects of three policy areas for future action 2008 by the RAND Corporation.
[31] Woods MS. How Communication Complicates the Patient Safety Movement. *Patient Safety and Quality Healthcare*, May/June 2006.
[32] Halverson AL, Casey JY, Andersson J, et al. Communication failure in the operating room. *Surgery.* 2011;149(3):305-10.
[33] Phillips DP, Barker GE. A July spike in fatal medication errors: a possible effect of new medical residents. *J Gen Intern Med.* 2010 Aug;25(8):774-9.
[34] Wu AW, Folkman S, McPhee SJ, et al. Do house officers learn from their mistakes? *JAMA.* 1991; 265(16):2089–94.
[35] Neale G, Woloshynowych M, Vincent C. Exploring the causes of adverse events in NHS hospital practice. *J. R. Soc. Med.* 2001; 94(7) 322–30.
[36] Ignaz Semmelweis. Wikipedia. http://en.wikipedia.org/wiki/Ignaz_ Semmelweis. Accessed July 31, 2012.

SECTION FOUR: CARDIOVASCULAR MEDICINE

In: Quality Improvement
Editors: K. W. Lobdell and S. C. Stamou
ISBN: 978-1-62417-390-5

Chapter 5

Quality Improvement in Cardiovascular Medicine: Challenges and Opportunities

Ziad Sergie and George D. Dangas
The Zena and Michael A. Wiener Cardiovascular Institute,
Mount Sinai Medical Center, One Gustave L. Levy Place,
New York, NY, US

Abstract

With the costs of healthcare delivery overwhelming the public and private sector in the United States, a focus on value, or the quality per dollar spent, has emerged in recent years.

Cardiovascular (CV) disease complexity, prevalence and mortality havedriven the practitioners of CV medicine to the forefront of quality improvement initiatives.

By applying some of the basic principles of quality assessment and improvement, professional societies and provider organizations in cardiology havedemonstrated leadership in advancing and disseminating the products of these efforts.

In this chapter, we will outlinethe major tools in quality improvement, and describe their application at the organizational and national levelsin order to achieve high-value care.

Introduction

The delivery of healthcare in the United States is fraught with significant gaps in quality, while the overall healthcare costs continue to rise, reaching 17.6% of US Gross Domestic Product (GDP) in 2010, or 2.6 trillion dollars.[1] Escalating costs exert a significant burden on the public and private sector, particularly in an economy that is recovering from the financial crisis and global recession of 2008. Slower growth in healthcare outlays has been evident in recent years; however spending increases are projected in 2014 with the expansion of medical coverage under the Affordable Care Act that was passed in 2010. [1] If the average growth rate of Medicare spending seen in recent decades is sustained, by 2060 almost all federal revenues will be spent on the Medicare program. [2] The growth in Medicare spending is projected to increase from 3.7% of GDP in 2011 to 5.7% of GDP in 2035, with an expected depletion of the Medicare Hospital Insurance Trust Fund by 2024.[3]Concordantly, innovation in biomedical sciences is under threat, because of reductions in healthcare-related governmental funding [4] and private capital (from venture capitalists and private equity groups), while the regulatory environment continues to be challenging. [5].

Healthcare expenditures on patients with cardiovascular (CV) disease constitute a major driver of overall healthcare costs,estimatedat $300 billion in 2008, [6] and expected to triple by 2030,[7] for a variety of reasons. Cardiovascular co-morbidities, including hypertension, hyperlipidemia, and coronary artery disease (CAD) are common chronic conditions, with high associated morbidity and mortality and increasing prevalence with age. It has recently been shown that the presence of only one or two traditional cardiovascular risk factors confers anincreasedlong-term risk of serious adverse outcomes.[8] Moreover, the incidence of acute stroke and acute myocardial infarction (AMI) is high, reaching 610000 new MIs annually and 795000 new or recurrent strokes.[6] Taking care of CV patients is expensive and often requires procedures (echocardiography, percutaneous coronary intervention (PCI), cardiac surgery), devices (pacemakers, implantable defibrillators), and specialized care (coronary care units, cardiology sub-specialists and ancillary services). Accordingly, CV disease was responsible for 16% of all healthcare expenditures in 2008.[6]

Many initiatives are underway that seek to bend the cost curve; however they are beyond the scope of this chapter. Our goal instead is to outline the major developments in quality improvement (QI) that have evolved in CV medical practice. In the first section, we will comment on the current environment of healthcare delivery, the perils of high variability in cardiac care, and some of the barriers to QI initiatives. We will then provide a practical definition of quality improvement with broad applicability, and discuss the three major tools of QI: clinical practice guidelines, performance measures, and appropriate use criteria. Afterwards, we will shift our focus to the concept of value in healthcare, and demonstrate common management practices of high-value organizations. Finally, we will discuss contemporary topics in CV medicine, such as the utilization of national CV registries in QI,the evolving principles of shared-decision making and patient-centered care, and the collaborative efforts to reduce CV disease burden nationwide.

The Current Landscape of Cardiovascular Medicine and Barriers to QI

Delivering care to patients with CV disease is usually a complicated and multidisciplinary process. These patients frequently have chronic conditions that require other specialists, such as diabetes and lung disease. They are often elderly and on a multitude of medications. They need close outpatient follow-up with a primary care physician and a cardiologist, and they are hospitalized frequently.

To add to the complexity, the field of CV medicine is evolving rapidly, with many high-quality clinical trials fine-tuning or even changing clinical practice. When the results of these trials are translated into clinical practice, patients typically experience improved outcomes. For example, mortality after AMI has declined in the past 5 decades, largely because of the widespread adoption of coronary care units, antiplatelet and anticoagulant therapy, coronary revascularization, and secondary prevention.[9]Reduction in AMI mortality from 1980 to

2000 has been accomplished by both control of CV risk factors and adoption of evidence-based treatments, where both aspects of care contributed equally to improved outcomes.[10]Yet despite these major advances, significant challenges to QI remain, some of which areshown in Figure 1.

The Dartmouth Atlas group was one of the first to highlight widespread geographical variability in the quality of care, primarily based on Medicare data that was analyzed according to hospital referral regions. They published the "Dartmouth Atlas of Cardiovascular Care" in 1999, which outlined significant regional variations in cardiovascular procedures in the US.

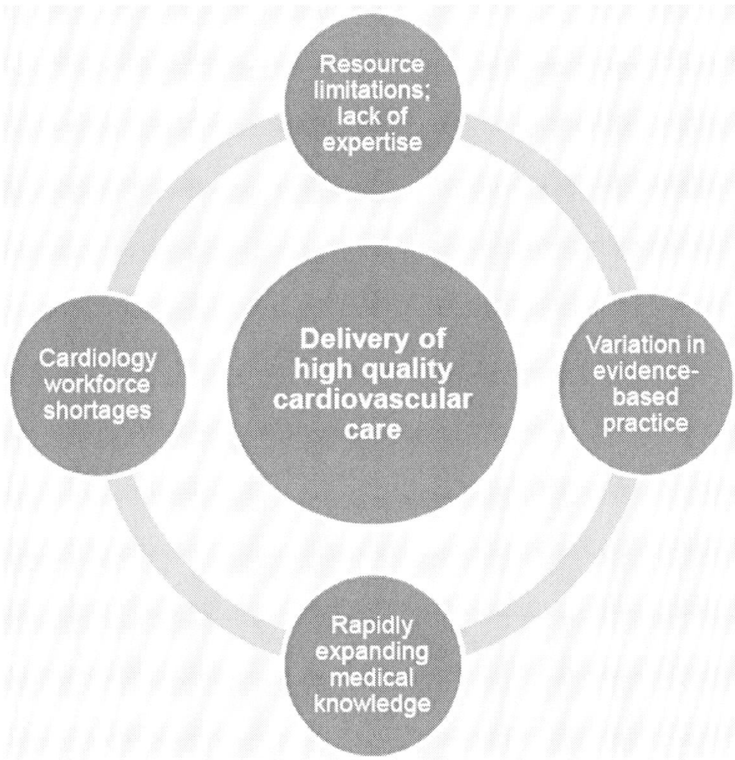
Resource limitations; lack of expertise
Delivery of high quality cardiovascular care
Cardiology workforce shortages
Variation in evidence-based practice
Rapidly expanding medical knowledge

Figure 1. Challenges to QI in the US.

These observations have been validated in a variety of healthcare delivery systems, [11] and in more contemporary populations. For example, an analysis of > 44 000 Medicare patients who presented with AMI between 1998 and 2001, found that regions that performed a higher volume of cardiac catheterizations were also more likely to do so for inappropriate or lower risk indications.[12] "Supply sensitive care" and "preference sensitive care" are the primary drivers of this variation, and higher intensity care is associated with similar or sometimes worse outcomes.[13] Therefore, one of the ultimate goals of QI initiatives is to reduce geographical differencesin care that cannot be explained by patient or clinical factors.

Another important challenge to high-quality care has been described in the literature, the "risk-treatment paradox." Numerous lines of clinical evidence have revealed that patientswhoare least likely to benefit from an intervention often receive it, while those most likely to benefit are undertreated. This lack of guideline adherence has been demonstrated in high risk patients with heart failure,[14]CAD, [15] and AMI.[16] Marso et al. recently provided another example of the "risk-treatment paradox" in patients who had undergone PCI. Bleeding rates and strategies to reduce bleeding were analyzed from the National Cardiovascular Data Registry (NCDR) involving > 1.5 million PCI patients from 2004 to 2008. The overall incidence of periprocedural bleeding was 2%, and while the use of both bivalirudin and vascular closure devices reduced bleeding the most in high-risk patients, they wereleast often used in this group (whereas manual compression was most used often in these high-risk patients).[17] This phenomenon is likely related to the confusing or conflicting lessons from trials and observational studies; however it also illustrates the importance of creating systems of care that disseminate the most up-to-date guidelines and validated risk stratification models to the bedside. The "risk-treatment paradox" has also been observed insituations where data is more limited and guidelines are based on expert opinion, such as patients presenting with AMI while on home warfarin therapy.[18]

Table 1. ACC recommendations to combat the cardiology workforce crisis

Problem	Recommendations
General cardiology supply shortage	Increase general fellowship positions. Allow for a delay in retirement; streamline the recertification process.
Future uncertainty of supply and demand	Systematically track supply / demand trends and publish results.
Need for practice efficiency	Support expansion of cardiology training programs for non-physician practitioners. Enhance the use of information technology and electronicmedical records.
Women under-representation in cardiology	Encourage work-life balance during fellowship and practice. Educate medical students and residents on the need for women in cardiology.
Black and Hispanic trainees less likely to specialize	Provide outreach programs and financial support to underrepresented minorities.
Underserved populations will be most affected by the impending cardiology shortage	Disseminate best and most efficient practices to these populations. Supportprograms that aim to provide CV care to these underserved patients.

Adding to these barriers, the US cardiology workforce is facing an impending shortage with respect to the supply needed. As described above, the need for CV specialists is clear, particularly as the advances in technology have made it difficult for generalists to step in and provide care for complex CV patients. The incidence of CV disease is projected to rise with an aging population, and the epidemics of obesity and metabolic syndrome. The estimated population growth of individuals > 65 years of age between 2010 and 2020 is 3.3% per year, while the average number of general cardiologists in 2008 per million was only 55.7.[19] Another study on hospital referral regions in patients > 65 years of age calculated a cardiology workforce growth rateof 19.2% between 1995 and 2007. [20] These discrepancies will most likely affect the underserved and rural areas in the US most severely. For these reasons, the American College of Cardiology (ACC) has set forth recommendations to address the workforce crisis, as summarized in Table 1.[19]

Defining Quality Improvement

Most definitions of QI rely on the concept of medical error reduction. In 1999, the Institute of Medicine (IOM) published their landmark report "To Err is Human" and estimated that up to 98000 lives are lost annually due to medical errors in hospitals.[21] The IOM also conceptualized quality care along six major domains to include "care that is safe, effective, patient-centered, timely, efficient, and equitable."[22]Following that report, the US Agency for Healthcare Research and Quality (AHRQ) saw significant increase in research funding, reaching $60 million in 2003.[23]The projected budget in 2011 for patient-centered health research was almost $252 million.[24]Similar to the IOM and AHRQ conceptions, other countries have relied on the same domains in their definition of quality care, which have a strong foundation in medical ethical principles of "justice, autonomy, beneficence and non-malfeasance."[25]

Another important framework identifies quality care as reduction of three types of errors, "underuse, overuse, or misuse."[26] Underuse is defined as failure to provide a service or treatment with known benefits to patients. This includes both therapeutic inertia (e.g. lack of up-titration of blood pressure medications for uncontrolled hypertension) and therapeutic nihilism (e.g. not prescribing an angiotensin-converting enzyme inhibitor for patients with systolic heart failure). Overuse is defined as providing care despite the lack of benefit to patients and the potential for harm, such as inappropriate cardiac surgeries or procedures. Misuse is when an appropriate treatment or service is provided, but an avoidable complication occurs obviating its benefit. Examples include any preventable complications of administered medications or surgical procedures, such as prescribing penicillin to a patient who needs it but is allergic to that antibiotic.

Despite these practical definitions, the process of measuring, monitoring, and promoting quality care is challenging, particularly in CV medical practice. In the following sections, we will describe three major tools of QI that have been developed and adopted by the cardiology community: clinical practice guidelines, performance measurement, and appropriate use criteria.

Clinical Practice Guidelines

One of the most effective tools to combat the widespread variability of quality care and to reduce the errors of misuse, overuse and underuse has been the development of clinical practice guidelines (CPGs). These guidelines are particularly useful given the rapid growthof medical knowledge and the large number of randomized clinical trials conducted in CV medicine every year. Their major function is to synthesize the available evidence into a clinically useful format, as recently described by the IOM: "CPGs are statements that include recommendations intended to optimize patient care that are informed by a systematic review of evidence and an assessment of the benefits and harms of alternative care options."[27]

The IOM also outlined some of the key aspects of "trustworthy guidelines" (Table 2). Accordingly, guidelines need to be developed by experts in the field based on high-quality systematic reviews, and they need to involve representative stakeholders including patients and patient representatives via a transparent process. Importantly, close attention to conflicts of interest need be made given their prevalence among panel members and committee chairmen, often undeclared.[28]

In the world of CV medicine, professional societies have taken a leadership role in developing CPGs, most notably the American College of Cardiology and American Heart Association (ACC/AHA). Initially developed for CV procedures in the 1980s, these guidelines have evolved to focus on a variety of specific conditions such as atrial fibrillation [29] and ST-elevation MI. [30, 31]Furthermore, CPGs form the basis for quality indicators, performance measurement, and appropriateness criteria.

Table 2. Standards for developing trustworthy guidelines according to the IOM

Standard	Recommendations
Transparency	The process of development and funding of a CPG should be available publicly
Management of conflict of interest	Needs to include written disclosures of all conflicts of interest, with potential divestment of financial investments relevant to the CPG; members with conflicts can be included in some circumstances, however not in chair or co-chair positions
Guideline development group composition	Should be multidisciplinary and balanced (patient and public involvement), with effective participation of all groups
Systematic reviews	Should meet the IOM standards for systematic reviews and comparative effectiveness research
Evidence foundations and strength of recommendations	Should explain the evidence for each recommendation, including any evidentiary gaps, the level of confidence, and the strength of each recommendation
Articulation of recommendations	Requires a standardized format, and strong recommendations should be worded appropriately
External review	Should be performed by the full spectrum of relevant stakeholders; a draft should also be made public prior to the final draft
Updating	Literature should be monitored regularly, and guidelines should be updated with new data that suggests a need to modify an existing recommendation

After synthesizing the available literature, the committee members come up with the most appropriate communication of their recommendations. The strength of each recommendation is graded as follows: Class I where the procedure/treatment is effective, Class IIa where weight of evidence is favorable, Class IIb where usefulness or efficacy is less well established, and Class III where the procedure/treatment is not useful or effective and may be harmful.[32] Level of evidence is also classified from Level A (derived from multiple randomized trials) to Level C (mostly expert opinion and consensus).

The end result of these efforts is a succinct summary of the totality of the evidence. One major limitation is that these documents frequently span many pages and are difficult to read. The ACC/AHA CPG task force has responded to this feedback from clinicians, and has been publishing clear tables that are easy to read and executive summaries of the key points. They also frequently publish focused updates that are shorter and incorporate the latest data from randomized trials. Many CPGs now include a convenient way to search for information within a document. Ultimately, therole of these CPGs is to strongly encourage clinicians to abide by Class I recommendations, and to provide consensus-based guidance for situations where data is limited, without supplanting clinical judgment. Guideline adherence, in turn, has been associated with improved patient outcomes including mortality after AMI.[33]Future guidelines need to follow the standards for trustworthy guidelines mentioned above, as these standards were recently reinforced by an international network of guideline developers.[34]

Performance Measurement

Well-formulated guidelines provide guidance to clinicians in their decision-making by synthesizing the available evidence. In order to ensure evidence-based healthcare delivery at the bedside, quality metricsthat are derived from Class I or III recommendations (mostly Level A) can be used to incentivize best practices. By quantifying adherence to these metrics, the quality of care can be measured and compared in a variety of settings. The process of developing theACC/AHA performance measures spansthree phases: building measurement sets, determining feasibility of measurement, and finally performance measurement.[35]In the first phase, the committee members define the target population and which dimension of care will be quantified, identify appropriate data sources, and build the performance measurement set. In the second phase,they evaluate the validity and reliability of each data item, and in the final phase they generate the output and determine whether data will be reported at the physician-level, group practice level, or health plan level. For example, the compliance with heart failure performance measures in 2010 as captured in three national registries is depicted in Figure 2.[6]

Close collaboration between guideline committee members and the performance measure task force is important, given that these guidelines are frequently updated to reflect the latest clinical trials.

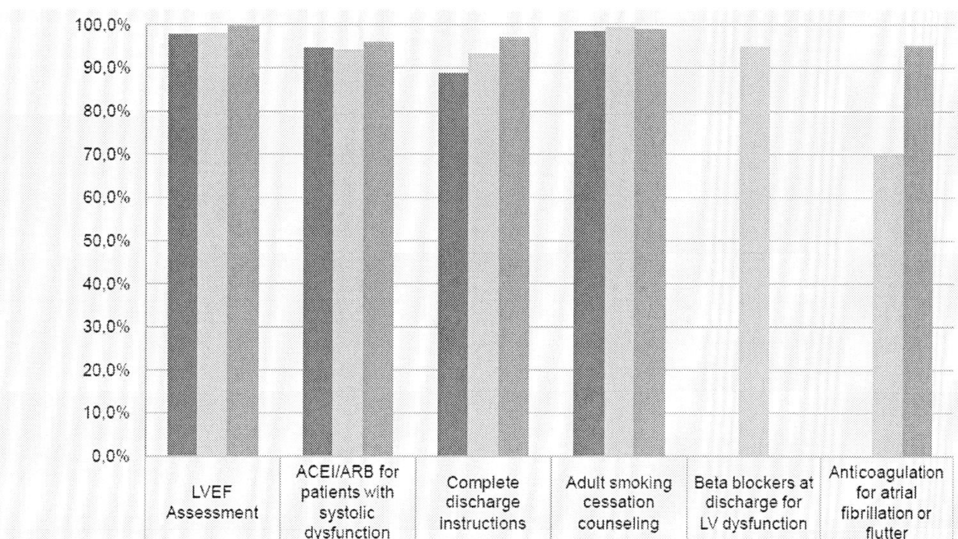

	LVEF Assessment	ACEI/ARB for patients with systolic dysfunction	Complete discharge instructions	Adult smoking cessation counseling	Beta blockers at discharge for LV dysfunction	Anticoagulation for atrial fibrillation or flutter
HIQR Program	97,8%	94,7%	88,9%	98,5%		
AHA GWTG-HF	98,0%	94,2%	93,3%	99,3%	94,8%	70,2%
VHA	100,0%	96,0%	97,0%	99,0%		95,0%

Reference: Circulation. 2012 Jan 3;125(1):e2-e220. Epub 2011 Dec 1.

Figure 2. Adherence to HF quality of care measures in 2010 in three registries.HIQR: Hospital Inpatient Quality Reporting; AHA GWTG-HF: American Heart Association's Get With The Guidelines – Heart Failure; VHA: Veterans Health Administration; LVEF: left ventricular ejection fraction; ACEI/ARB: angiotensin-converting enzyme inhibitor / angiotensin receptor blocker; LV: left ventricle.

One of the best known performance measures in CV medicine is the percentage of AMI patients who receive a beta blocker within 7 days of hospital discharge. This metric is based on the significant mortality reductions with beta blockers in this setting (up to 40% in various MI subgroups [36]), in addition to Class IB recommendations in the ACC/AHA guidelines. [37] First introduced in 1996, this evidence-based performance measurerallied the academic community, professional societies, health plans, and government agencies to allow system-wide change in healthcare delivery. As a product of these collaborations, almost all patients who present to a US hospital nowadays with AMI receive a beta blocker (compared with 34-38% in the mid-1990s), leading the National Committee for Quality Assurance to retire this measure altogether. [38] In other words, healthcare delivery in the US across settings has achieved reliability with respect to this performance measure.

Both the processes of care (e.g. aspirin in AMI, time to PCI) and patient outcomes (e.g. survival, cost, hospitalization) can be incorporated into performance measures documenting the quality of care. Governmental organizations and third party payers have been using these measures for two major initiatives: public reporting and pay-for-performance. Since 2007, the center for Medicare and Medicaid services (CMS) has been publishing data regarding hospital adherence to performance measures and 30-day risk-adjusted outcomes after AMI or heart failure in its "Hospital Compare" website.[39]Because of public availability, clinicians and patients can use this resource to engage in local quality assessment and improvement initiatives. Much work is still needed, however, as the optimal method to rank hospitals is still unclear. This was demonstrated in a comparison of different process and outcome measures in over 19000 patients from 153 hospitals, which found significant differences in hospital ranking depending on which measure was used.[40]Patients in particular should take note of the limitations of publicly available data, and should never delay seeking medical care in order to evaluate hospital rankings if they are acutely ill. Ranking is generally based on previous years' statistics, often lags for more than 1-2 years, and contains only limited data as reported. Therefore it is not designed to address decision-making questions regarding future treatment.

The CMS also relied on performance measures to develop a hospital pay-for-performance program, the Premier Hospital Quality Incentive demonstration. Early results appeared promising and demonstrated modest improvements in the processes of care among participant hospitals. [41] However, longer-term follow-up has cast doubts on the ability of pay-for-performance to improve patient outcomes. Most recently, the 252 hospitals that participated in the Premier demonstration were compared to 3363 hospitals that only provided public reporting (without pay-for-performance). Over 6 million patients were analyzed, and the 30-day mortality rate for AMI, heart failure, or pneumonia was not significantly different between the two hospital groups.[42] Despite these data, US hospitals will be reimbursed from Medicare based on their performance starting in October 2012, a major component of the Affordable Care Act that was signed into law in 2010. According to this program, also known as value-based purchasing, a percentage of reimbursement for each Diagnosis-Related Group will be at risk if hospitals do not abide by certain process measures.[43] Outcome measures (e.g. mortality) and hospital complications (e.g. acquired infections) will also be incorporated into this reimbursement model in 2014. The value-based purchasing formulas assign a score to both achievement and improvement in hospital quality, and newer formulas have been proposed that provide equitable distribution of payment scores across hospitals of varying socioeconomics and baseline performance. [44].

Appropriate Use Criteria

In recent years, there has been a significant increase in diagnostic testing and performed procedures in CV medicine. The overuse of such expensive modalities is critical, as demonstrated by the Dartmouth Atlas group. Furthermore, a recent systematic review of 172 studies found that overuse in general is limited to a small number of interventions and medications, mostly cardiovascular (including carotid endarterectomy, coronary angiography, and coronary artery bypass grafting). [45] By definition the appropriate use of diagnostic modalities and procedures excludes their underuse or misuse. In response to this widespread deficit in quality care, the ACC/AHA and other professional societies have developed another QI tool, the Appropriate Use Criteria (AUC). These AUCs rely on the guidelines and clinical evidence in order to evaluate clinical scenarios where a patient may benefit or be harmed from a test or intervention. Thus AUCs can help assess variability in healthcare services and utilization patterns of care that most likely do not benefit patients.

In 2009, the ACC/AHA published the AUC for coronary revascularization. Because PCI is a common procedure in the US (almost 600000 per year) with associated costs and potential harms to patients, it presents an important opportunity for improving efficiency and value in healthcare delivery. The process of developing AUC first requires a writing committee to come up with specific patient scenarios. A separate technical panel, composed of a diverse group of professionals (mostly physician experts), assigns a score to each indication from 1 (least appropriate) to 9 (most appropriate). From the median of individual ratings, each clinical scenario is classified as appropriate (score of 7-9), uncertain (score of 4-6), or inappropriate (score of 1-3).[46] The ACC/AHA used the following definition of AUC for PCI: "coronary revascularization is appropriate when the expected benefits, in terms of survival or health outcomes (symptoms, functional status, and/or quality of life) exceed the expected negative consequences of the procedure."[46]

Based on these criteria, Chan et al. analyzed data from close to 1100 US hospitals that reported their data on over 500000 PCIs to the National Cardiovascular Data Registry (NCDR). They divided PCIs into acute or non-acute groups, and determined the percentage in each AUC category. In the acute PCI group, 98.6% of PCIs were classified as appropriate; whereas in the non-acute group, 38% were classified as uncertain and 11.6% as inappropriate.[47] Moreover, there was substantial hospital variation in the non-acute group. Over 95% of patients who underwent PCI characterized as inappropriate were not treated with optimal medical therapy,[47] despite recent trials that have shown a similar impact on patient outcomes when compared with revascularization in stable patients.[48]

This analysis has several limitations that were summarized by Marso et al.[49], and they pertain to AUC in general. First of all, the PCI AUC committee was composed of 17 members but only 4 members had expertise in PCI. While this was done to limit financial conflicts of interest and other forms of bias, it may have decreased the accuracy of the AUC Technical Panel. For example, when comparing the appropriateness ratings for 68 PCI indications determined by the AUC Technical Panel and 85 clinical cardiologists, the overall concordance was 84%.[50] However, there was only modest agreement (70%) on the inappropriate indications, with significant variation among individual physicians. Second, the AUC criteria for PCI in the non-acute setting were dependent on pre-procedural stress testing, which lacks specific guidelines and is largely dependent on the NCDR abstractors to interpret (who in turn have varying levels of expertise). Furthermore, Fractional Flow Reserve data were not incorporated in these algorithms, recently shown to be predictive of future cardiac events in patients with multivessel coronary disease.[51]Finally, unusual clinical scenarios (e.g. cardiac workup pre-transplantation of a solid organ) have not been part of the AUC either. A focused update on these AUC for coronary revascularization was recently published to address some of these concerns.[52]Moving forward, AUC will require validation and proof that appropriate care actually benefits patients or vice versa. Of note, a recent NCDR analysis failed to demonstrate a significant association between the proportion of inappropriate PCIs at each hospital andworse clinical outcomes including in-hospital mortality, bleeding, or quality of discharge.[53]Addressing these limitations will improve the accuracy and applicability of future AUC, particularly as they gain widespread application to other CV technologies.[54]

Delivering High-Value Care

Healthcare delivery in the US is undergoing a significant transformation, from small autonomous entities (e.g. physician offices) with minimal integration and variable care to larger integrated groups that rely on standardization and performance measurement. The tools of QI are playing a key role in this transformation and emphasis on value. Defined by Swensen et al., the value of health care depends on "its design (the right treatment for the right patient at the right time), its execution (reliably doing it right every time to achieve the best outcomes), and its cost." [55]Likewise, the value of any intervention is best defined as the ratio of overall benefit to cost, anda practical framework for assessing the value of interventions was recently described by Owens et al.[56]In their formulation, the benefits and harms of each intervention need to be assessed a priori and the costs need to include both the upfront intervention costs and any spending that occurs downstream. Value can then be assessed by calculating the "incremental cost-effectiveness ratio or cost per quality-adjusted life year (QALY) gained," with a generally accepted threshold of $30 000 to $50 000 per QALY.[56]

The goal of such calculations is to eliminatethose interventions that provide no benefit, and to promote those that increase value. Overuse and overtreatment reduction are crucial to eliminating overall waste in healthcare spending, butthere are many other aspects of care that provide little value. Berwick et al. postulated that six categories of waste contribute 21%-34% of all spending depending on lower or midpoint estimates: failure of care delivery, lack of coordination, overtreatment, complexity of administration, pricing failures, and fraud/abuse.[57] Physicians and provider organizations need to play a major role in improving the value of healthcare, and can do so by reducing unnecessary care, preventable errors (such as healthcare associated infections) and process inefficiency.[58]Notably, a focus on specific efficiency metrics(thatevaluate resource allocation)is gaining traction, and the ACC/AHA has already outlined some of their most important attributes as they pertain to public reporting and provider comparisons.[59]

Based on these principles, an insightful framework for characterizing high-value organizations was recently proposed. The following four aspects were highlighted: "specification and planning, infrastructure and design, measurement and oversight, and self-study."[60] These four "habits" are systematic practices by high-value organizations at all times thatmay be transferable to other organizations seeking to improve quality of care.[60]To evaluate aspects of organizational culture more closely, Curry et al. performed a qualitative survey of 158 hospital staff members involved in AMI care at 11 hospitals, and found significant differences in organizational factors between the top and bottom performing hospitalsvis-à-vis AMI mortality rates.[61]These features included organizational values, senior management involvement, communication, and problem solving. The same research group performed a cross-sectional survey of 537 hospitals and found several organizational factors that were associated with reduced AMI mortality. These included monthly meetings between clinicians and staff involved in transporting patients to the hospital, a culture of creative problem-solving, physician and nurse champions for quality of care, onsite cardiologists, and intensive care nurses that did not work in the catheterization laboratory.[62] Both studies elucidate some of the management features that can be promoted at the organizational level to improve AMI outcomes and quality of care.

Certain provider organizations have demonstrated leadership and success in improving the value of care delivery. Key to their success is the process of organizational restructuring and systems engineering in order to promote a culture of high-value care. For example, the Mayo Clinic has a standardized "value creation system" composed of the following four key phases applied throughout the organization: alignmentand prioritization of resources, discovery, diffusion of best practices, and consistent measurement.[63] Likewise, continuous quality improvement programs have been implemented in the cardiac catheterization laboratory [64, 65] and in the setting of cardiac surgery.[66] These concepts are being translated from other industries to healthcare with promising results, as seen with the application of the Toyota production system to cardiac surgery.[67] The Intermountain Healthcare System has also been a leader in reducing the costs of healthcare by promoting quality assessment and improvement.[68] In order to promote such collaborations, there is now momentum towards aligning payment incentives for providers with thereliable delivery of high-value care.[69]

Data Collection, Registries, and Real-World Collaborations

Consistent definitions thatdescribe patient management decisions and outcomes arecrucial for all QI initiatives. These standardized benchmarks allow appropriate comparisons across clinical trials and observational studies, and are particularly useful when conducting meta-analyses and systematic reviews.

The ACC/AHA has created a task force on clinical data standards in order to facilitate cross comparisons between studies, to enable the development of representative registries, and to ultimately form the basis of electronic medical records.[70] In the field of interventional cardiology, such data standards have been particularly important with regards to AMI and PCI. Given the critical association between bleeding and adverse outcomes, [71] for example, the heterogeneity of bleeding definitions is a hindrance to accurate comparison of antithrombotic and invasive strategies. Therefore, the Bleeding Academic Research Consortium representatives have created a new definition of bleeding that has wide applicability and is heavily reliant on event adjudication.[72]

Moving from data standards to data collection, the ACC demonstrated leadershipby lauchingone of the most comprehensive registries in the USin 1997, the national cardiovacular data registry (NCDR).[73]Almost 2200 hospitals in the US currently participate in this data repository, and they receive quarterly and annual reports on quality-of-care and outcomes performance. The NCDR has expanded from the CathPCI registry to cover carotid artery procedures (CARE), implantable defibrillators (ICD), congenital heart disease (IMPACT), and outpatient care (PINNACLE), as listed in Table 3. The ACTION Get with the Guidelines (GWTG) registry is a merged dataset between the AHA GWTG web-based registry for AMI QI [74] and the ACC ACTION registry. By May 2010, 383 hospitals have participated and over 140000 records have been submitted to this registry, with only 5% of fields with missing data.[75]These registries provide important insights on adherence to guidelines, variation in clinical practice, and overall patient outcomes including mortality. For example, an analysis from the PINNACLE ambulatory care registry involving 27 US clinical practice sites showed only moderate compliance with ACC/AHA performance measures for CAD and heart failure, with significant inter-site variation.[76] Linking data from these registries with claims data from third party payers has enabled prediction models and comparative effectiveness analyses on coronary revascularization in Medicare patients.[77-79]Moreover, participation in high-quality data registries is mandatory for governmental reimbursement for carotid stenting [80] and for transcatheter aortic valve replacement [81]; conversely this is not a reimbursement requirement for the surgical treatment of carotid or aortic stenosis.

Table 3. NCDR Registries

Registry	Patient Population
ACTION - GWTG	A national AMI surveillance system, which incorporates the ACC/AHA performance measures and the class I recommendations of the ACC/AHA clinical practice guidelines
CARE	Assesses carotid artery stenting and endarterectomy procedures, regardless of which specialty performs the procedure; includes calculation of NIH stroke scale
CathPCI	Includes cardiac disease patients who receive diagnostic catheterization and / or percutaneous coronary intervention procedures
ICD	Helps participating hospitals measure and improve care for patients receiving implantable cardiac defibrillators
IMPACT	Collects data and outcomes on pediatric and adult congenital disease patients who undergo cardiac catheterization
STS / ACC TVT	Collaboration between STS and ACC to track data and outcomes on patients who undergo transcatheter aortic valve replacement
PINNACLE	Captures data related to outpatient care for coronary artery disease, heart failure, and atrial fibrillation

Reference: http://www.ncdr.com/webncdr/common/; accessed May 22, 2012.

ACTION – GWTG: Acute Coronary Treatment and Intervention Outcomes Network - Get with the guidelines; CARE: Carotid Artery Revascularization and Endarterectomy; CathPCI: Diagnostic Catheterization and Percutaneous Coronary Intervention; ICD: Implantable Cardiac Defibrillator; IMPACT: Improving Pediatric and Adult Congenital Treatment; STS / ACC TVT: Society of Thoracic Surgeons / American College of Cardiology Transcatheter Valve Replacement); PINNACLE: Practice Innovation and Clinical Excellence.

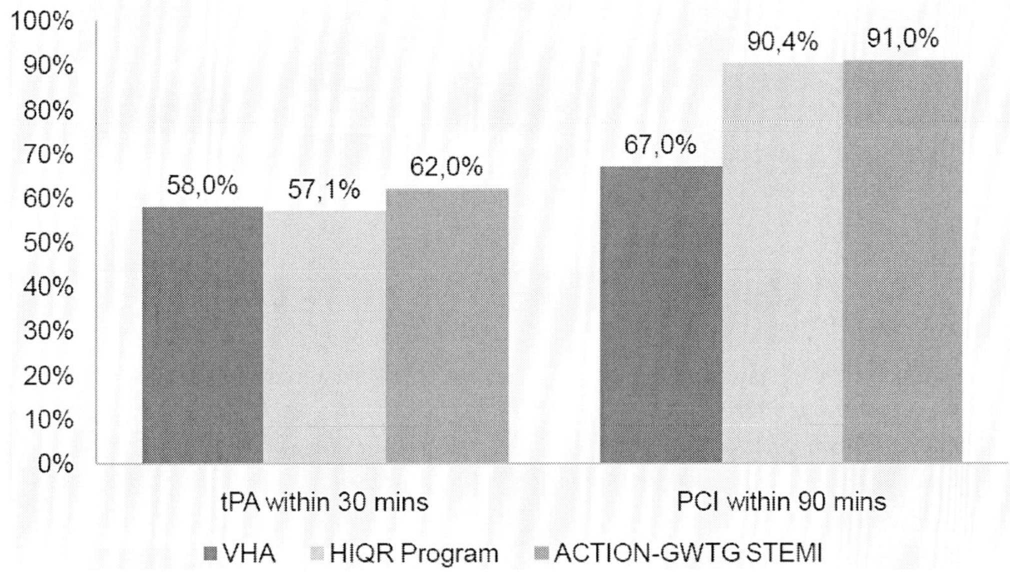

Reference: Circulation. 2012 Jan 3;125(1):e2-e220. Epub 2011 Dec 1.

Figure 3. Performance according to reperfusion metrics for ACS in 2010. ACS: acute coronary syndrome; VHA: Veterans Health Administration; HIQR: Hospital Inpatient Quality Reporting; ACTION-GWTG: Acute Coronary Treatment and Intervention Outcomes Registry –Get With The Guidelines; STEMI: ST-elevation myocardial infarction; tPA: tissue-type plasminogen activator.

Building on these efforts, several collaborations have occurred nationwide to improve the quality of care. The door-to-balloon coalition is an important example and should be considered a model for medical practice improvement nationwide.

It was initiated in 2006 as an alliance between the ACC and 38 other organizations, with the goal of reducing door-to-balloon times for patients presenting with STEMI to ≤ 90 minutes, according to contemporary guidelines. Based on data from the NCDR CathPCI registry, improvement was seen in door-to-balloon time, from 52.5% to 76.4% over a three period, with correlated increases in compliance with important process measures. [82]

Restructuring the systems of STEMI care to enable reliable compliance with key process measures was the most important determinant of sustainable decreases in door-to-balloon time, as demonstrated by the Mayo Clinic STEMI protocol. [83] Factors that are crucial include emergency room activation of the catheterization laboratory with a single call, staff arrival within 30 minutes,and prompt performance feedback to ensure continuous improvement and inter-department communication. As shown in Figure 3, greater than 90% of patients in 2010 hadattained the door-to-balloon time goal of ≤ 90minutes in two major national registries. [6]

In 2011, the Department of Health and Human Services launched the "Million Hearts" initiative, another important collaborative effort for QI involving the AHA and many other organizations. The goal of this initiative is to "prevent 1million heart attacks and strokes over the next 5 years."[84] This will require two major categories of intervention: improving the management of the "ABCS" (including Aspirin when appropriate, Blood pressure control, Cholesterol management, and Smoking cessation), and expanding community prevention efforts. The focus on the "ABCS" is based on a recent survey of US adult data (over the age of 20 years), where 49.7% (or over 107 million) adults had at least one of these three risk factors.[85] Improvement in clinical management of the "ABCS" will be facilitated by their incorporation into performance metrics and electronic medical record meaningful use criteria, in addition to a pharmacist led campaign.[84] The "Million Hearts" initiative will also facilitate prevention efforts by expanding policies and programs to reduce tobacco-use, sodium intake and trans fat food content. Of note, full implementation of the Affordable Care Act of 2010 will help these initiativesby expanding medical coverage and proposing cost-savings for patients who seek preventative care.[84]

Focus on Patient-Centered Care

Thus far in this chapter, we have described the important tools of quality improvement and their applications in the field of cardiology. In this section we will focus on one of the fundamental aspects of healthcare delivery: the process of clinical decision-making and the doctor-patient relationship. Considerable progress has been made in this field, including a reformulation of informed consent via the evolving conception of "shared decision-making." Central to this concept is the requirement that physicians take into account patient preferences and values when offering alternative treatment options and interventions. The healthcare system in the US is generally shifting towards patient-centeredness as a defining aspect of quality care, reflecting one of the six major goals elaborated in the 2001 IOM report.[86]Moreover, in addition to process and outcome measures, the metrics for quality assessment in the future will likely include "goal-directed, patient-centered decision making."[87]

For most clinical decisions in the field of cardiology, there are multiple reasonable management options. Shared decision-making with patients can be accomplished by completing the following three tasks: "estimating patients' outcomes as a function of their individual risks, defining these outcomes as a function of alternative treatments, and sharing this information with patients in a manner they understand."[88]Patient-specific risk scores are vitalto the first two tasks, and are particularly useful in the peri-procedural setting. For example, Mehran et al. previously published a risk score for post-PCI contrast-induced nephropathy that includes eight readily available patient and procedural characteristics.[89] Likewise, a post-PCI bleeding risk score was formulated from pooling data from three large randomized trials that enrolled a spectrum of CAD patients.[71]An analysis from Harmonizing Outcomes with Revascularization and Stents in Acute Myocardial Infarction (HORIZONS-AMI) trial revealed the individual predictors of stent thrombosis, and the protective effects of pre-randomization heparin and high-dose clopidogrel in this setting.[90] Finally, the predictors of mortality following AMI are currently being analyzed from the HORIZONS-AMI trial. These efforts are fundamental to individualized risk assessment, and the process of communicating these risks has been studied extensively, as illustrated in asystematic review of 86 studies on decision aideffectiveness in various clinical settings.[91]Ultimately, shared decision-making is most appropriate in the non-acute setting where there are clear management alternatives;as mentioned above, it is an evolution of informed consent. [92, 93].

Considerable research efforts are currently being devoted to these innovations in care deliveryas they have the potential to significantly change clinical practice. For example, the standard of care for low-risk patients presenting to the emergency with chest pain is to evaluate for cardiac injury and to perform risk stratification for ischemic heart disease(usually via stress testing), as articulated by the AHA guidelines.[94] Hess et al. applied the concepts of shared decision-making to this common clinical scenario, and randomized 204 low-risk patients to a decision aid (a diagram clearly displaying the pre-test probability of AMI and the available management options) or usual care. After each encounter, the patients in the decision aid group demonstrated greater knowledge transfer and engagement in decision-making and were less likely to choose to be admitted for stress testing; there were no adverse cardiac events in either group at 30-day follow-up.[95]These studies are important because they demonstrate the power of shared decision-making in aligning patient preferences with appropriate resource utilization. The most recent advanced heart failure guidelines from the AHA advocate such a patient-centered approach.[96]

Notably, the concepts of patient-centered care are highly influential on contemporary public policy in the US. For example, the Affordable Care Act of 2010 has allocated funding for a separate Patient-Centered Outcomes Research Institute, in order to advance comparative effectiveness studies.[97, 98]It has also established the Medicare Shared Savings program as a foundation for patient-centered accountable care organizations.[99] This realignment of reimbursement models has the potential to improve coordination of care between primary physicians and specialists, thus potentially improving quality and lowering costs. Another evolving model of care delivery is the patient-centered medical home or health home. Given that a small percentage of patients account for the majority of health expenditures, advances in care that focus on these patients are necessary, such asthe proposed well-coordinated "health improvement communities."[100] Similarly, a recent survey of complex patients in eleven countries (including the US) found a widespread lack of care coordination, while practices with features of a typical medical home delivered higher quality care.[101]These models of care delivery will become the standard of care, and may play a major role in improving the value of healthcare delivery in the US.

Conclusion

Despite the difficulty in predicting the upcoming regulatory environment in the US, a focus on quality and value in healthcare delivery is inevitable and will be an integral part of future care delivery models. Ultimately, we owe it to our patients to strive for safe, effective, standardized care, that also takes into account their preferences and values. Achieving these goals will requireclose attentiontothe cost and value of various cardiovascular treatments and interventions as well as performance measurement and shared decision-making. Healthcare providers in general and cardiology practitioners in particular have an opportunity to take a leadership role in these initiatives, in order to improvecardiovascular health for individuals and populations.

References

[1] Keehan, S.P., et al., National health spending projections through 2020: economic recovery and reform drive faster spending growth. *Health affairs,* 2011. 30(8): p. 1594-605.

[2] White, C. and P.B. Ginsburg, Slower growth in Medicare spending--is this the new normal? *The New England Journal of Medicine*, 2012. 366(12): p. 1073-5.

[3] Social Security and Medicare Boards of Trustees. *Status of the Social Security and Medicare Programs.* http://www.socialsecurity.gov/ OACT/TRSUM/index.html. Accessed: April 23, 2012 2012.
[4] Fuster, V., et al., Academic careers in cardiovascular medicine. *Circulation,* 2009. 119(5): p. 754-60.
[5] Edelman, E.R. and M.B. Leon, The fiber of modern society. *Science translational medicine,* 2011. 3(89): p. 89cm14.
[6] Roger, V.L., et al., Heart disease and stroke statistics--2012 update: a report from the american heart association. *Circulation*, 2012. 125(1): p. e2-e220.
[7] Heidenreich, P.A., et al., Forecasting the future of cardiovascular disease in the United States: a policy statement from the American Heart Association. *Circulation,* 2011. 123(8): p. 933-44.
[8] Berry, J.D., et al., Lifetime risks of cardiovascular disease. The New England journal of medicine, 2012. 366(4): p. 321-9.
[9] Nabel, E.G. and E. Braunwald, A tale of coronary artery disease and myocardial infarction. *The New England Journal of Medicine,* 2012. 366(1): p. 54-63.
[10] Ford, E.S., et al., Explaining the decrease in U.S. deaths from coronary disease, 1980-2000. *The New England Journal of Medicine*, 2007. 356(23): p. 2388-98.
[11] Ko, D.T., et al., Regional differences in process of care and outcomes for older acute myocardial infarction patients in the United States and Ontario, Canada. *Circulation,* 2007. 115(2): p. 196-203.
[12] Ko, D.T., et al., Regional variation in cardiac catheterization appropriateness and baseline risk after acute myocardial infarction. *Journal of the American College of Cardiology*, 2008. 51(7): p. 716-23.
[13] Wennberg, J.E., Time to tackle unwarranted variations in practice. *British Medical Journal*, 2011. 342.
[14] Lee, D.S., et al., Risk-treatment mismatch in the pharmacotherapy of heart failure.*JAMA: the Journal of the American Medical Association,* 2005. 294(10): p. 1240-7.
[15] McAlister, F.A., et al., Exploring the treatment-risk paradox in coronary disease. *Archives of internal medicine*, 2007. 167(10): p. 1019-25.
[16] Roe, M.T., et al., The influence of risk status on guideline adherence for patients with non-ST-segment elevation acute coronary syndromes. *American Heart Journal,* 2006. 151(6): p. 1205-13.
[17] Marso, S.P., et al., Association between use of bleeding avoidance strategies and risk of periprocedural bleeding among patients undergoing percutaneous coronary intervention. *JAMA: the Journal of the American Medical Association,* 2010. 303(21): p. 2156-64.
[18] Subherwal, S., et al., Admission International Normalized Ratio Levels, Early Treatment Strategies, and Major Bleeding Risk Among Non-ST-Segment-Elevation Myocardial Infarction Patients on Home Warfarin Therapy: Insights From the National Cardiovascular Data Registry. *Circulation,* 2012. 125(11): p. 1414-23.
[19] Rodgers, G.P., et al., ACC 2009 survey results and recommendations: Addressing the cardiology workforce crisis A report of the ACC board of trustees workforce task force. *Journal of the American College of Cardiology,* 2009. 54(13): p. 1195-208.

[20] Aneja, S., et al., US cardiologist workforce from 1995 to 2007: modest growth, lasting geographic maldistribution especially in rural areas. *Health affairs*, 2011. 30(12): p. 2301-9.

[21] Medicine, I.o., *To Err is Human: Building a Safer Health System.* Washington DC: National Academy Press, 2001.

[22] Medicine, I.o., *Crossing the quality chasm: a new health system for the 21st century.* Washington DC: National Academy Press, 2001.

[23] Meyer, G.S., et al., The US Agency for Healthcare Research and Quality's activities in patient safety research. *International Journal for Quality in Health Care*, 2003. 15: p. I25-I30.

[24] AHRQ. Budget Estimates for Appropriations Committees, *Fiscal Year* 2011. http://www.ahrq.gov/about/cj2011/cjweb11over.htm; Accessed April 4, 2012.

[25] Atkinson, S., et al., Defining quality and quality improvement. *Clinical medicine,* 2010. 10(6): p. 537-9.

[26] Chassin, M.R. and R.W. Galvin, The urgent need to improve health care quality. Institute of Medicine National Roundtable on Health Care Quality. *JAMA: the Journal of the American Medical Association,* 1998. 280(11): p. 1000-5.

[27] Medicine, I.o. *Clinical Practice Guidelines We can Trust.*www.iom.edu/cpgstandards; Accessed April 4, 2012 2011.

[28] Neuman, J., et al., Prevalence of financial conflicts of interest among panel members producing clinical practice guidelines in Canada and United States: cross sectional study. *BMJ,* 2011. 343: p. d5621.

[29] Fuster, V., et al., 2011 ACCF/AHA/HRS focused updates incorporated into the ACC/AHA/ESC 2006 guidelines for the management of patients with atrial fibrillation: a report of the American College of Cardiology Foundation/American Heart Association Task Force on practice guidelines. *Circulation,* 2011. 123(10): p. e269-367.

[30] Gibbons, R.J., S.C. Smith, Jr., and E. Antman, American College of Cardiology/American Heart Association clinical practice guidelines: Part II: evolutionary changes in a continuous quality improvement project. *Circulation*, 2003. 107(24): p. 3101-7.

[31] Kushner, F.G., et al., 2009 Focused Updates: ACC/AHA Guidelines for the Management of Patients With ST-Elevation Myocardial Infarction (updating the 2004 Guideline and 2007 Focused Update) and ACC/AHA/SCAI Guidelines on Percutaneous Coronary Intervention (updating the 2005 Guideline and 2007 Focused Update): a report of the American College of Cardiology Foundation/American Heart Association Task Force on Practice Guidelines. *Circulation,* 2009. 120(22): p. 2271-306.

[32] Gibbons, R.J., S. Smith, and E. Antman, American College of Cardiology/American Heart Association clinical practice guidelines: Part I: where do they come from? *Circulation,* 2003. 107(23): p. 2979-86.

[33] Peterson, E.D., et al., Association between hospital process performance and outcomes among patients with acute coronary syndromes. *JAMA: the Journal of the American Medical Association,* 2006. 295(16): p. 1912-20.

[34] Qaseem, A., et al., Guidelines International Network: Toward International Standards for Clinical Practice Guidelines. *Annals of internal medicine,* 2012. 156(7): p. 525-531.

[35] Spertus, J.A., et al., American College of Cardiology and American Heart Association methodology for the selection and creation of performance measures for quantifying the quality of cardiovascular care. *Circulation,* 2005. 111(13): p. 1703-12.

[36] Gottlieb, S.S., R.J. McCarter, and R.A. Vogel, Effect of beta-blockade on mortality among high-risk and low-risk patients after myocardial infarction. *The New England Journal of Medicine*, 1998. 339(8): p. 489-97.

[37] Anderson, J.L., et al., 2011 ACCF/AHA Focused Update Incorporated Into the ACC/AHA 2007 Guidelines for the Management of Patients With Unstable Angina/Non-ST-Elevation Myocardial Infarction: a report of the American College of Cardiology Foundation/American Heart Association Task Force on Practice Guidelines. *Circulation,* 2011. 123(18): p. e426-579.

[38] Lee, T.H., Eulogy for a quality measure. *The New England Journal of Medicine,* 2007. 357(12): p. 1175-7.

[39] Krumholz, H.M. and S.L. Normand, Public reporting of 30-day mortality for patients hospitalized with acute myocardial infarction and heart failure. *Circulation,* 2008. 118(13): p. 1394-7.

[40] Hernandez, A.F., et al., The need for multiple measures of hospital quality: results from the Get with the Guidelines-Heart Failure Registry of the American Heart Association. *Circulation*, 2011. 124(6): p. 712-9.

[41] Lindenauer, P.K., et al., Public reporting and pay for performance in hospital quality improvement. *The New England Journal of Medicine,* 2007. 356(5): p. 486-96.

[42] Jha, A.K., et al., The long-term effect of premier pay for performance on patient outcomes. *The New England Journal of Medicine,* 2012. 366(17): p. 1606-15.

[43] Ryan, A. and J. Blustein, Making the best of hospital pay for performance. *The New England Journal of Medicine*, 2012. 366(17): p. 1557-9.

[44] Borden, W.B. and J. Blustein, Valuing improvement in value-based purchasing. Circulation. *Cardiovascular quality and outcomes*, 2012. 5(2): p. 163-70.

[45] Korenstein, D., et al., Overuse of health care services in the United States: an understudied problem. *Archives of internal medicine,* 2012. 172(2): p. 171-8.

[46] Patel, M.R., et al., ACCF/SCAI/STS/AATS/AHA/ASNC 2009 Appropriateness Criteria for Coronary Revascularization: a report by the American College of Cardiology Foundation Appropriateness Criteria Task Force, Society for Cardiovascular Angiography and Interventions, Society of Thoracic Surgeons, American Association for Thoracic Surgery, American Heart Association, and the American Society of Nuclear Cardiology Endorsed by the American Society of Echocardiography, the Heart Failure Society of America, and the Society of Cardiovascular Computed Tomography. *Journal of the American College of Cardiology,* 2009. 53(6): p. 530-53.

[47] Chan, P.S., et al., Appropriateness of percutaneous coronary intervention. *JAMA: the Journal of the American Medical Association,* 2011. 306(1): p. 53-61.

[48] Borden, W.B., et al., Patterns and intensity of medical therapy in patients undergoing percutaneous coronary intervention. *JAMA: the Journal of the American Medical Association,* 2011. 305(18): p. 1882-9.

[49] Marso, S.P., et al., Percutaneous coronary intervention use in the United States: defining measures of appropriateness. JACC. *Cardiovascular interventions,* 2012. 5(2): p. 229-35.

[50] Chan, P.S., et al., Concordance of physician ratings with the appropriate use criteria for coronary revascularization. *Journal of the American College of Cardiology,* 2011. 57(14): p. 1546-53.

[51] Tonino, P.A., et al., Angiographic versus functional severity of coronary artery stenoses in the FAME study fractional flow reserve versus angiography in multivessel evaluation. *Journal of the American College of Cardiology,* 2010. 55(25): p. 2816-21.

[52] Patel, M.R., et al., ACCF/SCAI/STS/AATS/AHA/ASNC/HFSA/SCCT 2012 Appropriate use criteria for coronary revascularization focused update: a report of the American College of Cardiology Foundation Appropriate Use Criteria Task Force, Society for Cardiovascular Angiography and Interventions, Society of Thoracic Surgeons, American Association for Thoracic Surgery, American Heart Association, American Society of Nuclear Cardiology, and the Society of Cardiovascular Computed Tomography. *Journal of the American College of Cardiology,* 2012. 59(9): p. 857-81.

[53] Bradley, S.M., et al., Hospital Percutaneous Coronary Intervention Appropriateness and In-Hospital Procedural Outcomes: Insights From the NCDR. Circulation. *Cardiovascular quality and outcomes*, 2012. 5(3): p. 290-7.

[54] Bonow, R.O., et al., ACCF/AHA methodology for the development of quality measures for cardiovascular technology: a report of the American College of Cardiology Foundation/American Heart Association Task Force on Performance Measures. *Circulation,* 2011. 124(13): p. 1483-502.

[55] Swensen, S.J., et al., Cottage industry to postindustrial care--the revolution in health care delivery. *The New England Journal of Medicine,* 2010. 362(5): p. e12.

[56] Owens, D.K., et al., High-value, cost-conscious health care: concepts for clinicians to evaluate the benefits, harms, and costs of medical interventions. *Annals of internal medicine*, 2011. 154(3): p. 174-80.

[57] Berwick, D.M. and A.D. Hackbarth, Eliminating Waste in US Health Care. JAMA : the journal of the American Medical Association, 2012.

[58] Swensen, S.J., et al., Controlling healthcare costs by removing waste: what American doctors can do now. *BMJ quality and safety*, 2011. 20(6): p. 534-7.

[59] Krumholz, H.M., et al., Standards for measures used for public reporting of efficiency in health care: a scientific statement from the American Heart Association Interdisciplinary Council on Quality of Care and Outcomes Research and the American College of Cardiology Foundation. *Circulation*, 2008. 118(18): p. 1885-93.

[60] Bohmer, R.M., The four habits of high-value health care organizations. *The New England journal of medicine*, 2011. 365(22): p. 2045-7.

[61] Curry, L.A., et al., What distinguishes top-performing hospitals in acute myocardial infarction mortality rates? A qualitative study. *Annals of internal medicine,* 2011. 154(6): p. 384-90.

[62] Bradley, E.H., et al., Hospital strategies for reducing risk-standardized mortality rates in acute myocardial infarction. *Annals of internal medicine,* 2012. 156(9): p. 618-26.

[63] Swensen, S.J., et al., The mayo clinic value creation system. *American Journal of medical quality: the official Journal of the American College of Medical Quality,* 2012. 27(1): p. 58-65.

[64] Brindis, R.G. and G.J. Dehmer, Continuous quality improvement in the cardiac catheterization laboratory: are the benefits worth the cost and effort? *Circulation,* 2006. 113(6): p. 767-70.

[65] Moscucci, M., et al., Association of a continuous quality improvement initiative with practice and outcome variations of contemporary percutaneous coronary interventions. *Circulation,* 2006.113(6):p.814-22.
[66] Stamou, S.C., et al., Continuous quality improvement program and major morbidity after cardiac surgery. *The American Journal of cardiology,* 2008. 102(6): p. 772-7.
[67] Culig, M.H., et al., Improving patient care in cardiac surgery using Toyota production system based methodology. *The Annals of thoracic surgery,* 2011. 91(2): p. 394-9.
[68] James, B.C. and L.A. Savitz, How Intermountain trimmed health care costs through robust quality improvement efforts. *Health affairs*, 2011. 30(6): p. 1185-91.
[69] McMahon, L.F., Jr. and V. Chopra, Health care cost and value: the way forward. *JAMA: the Journal of the American Medical Association,* 2012. 307(7): p. 671-2.
[70] Radford, M.J., et al., ACC/AHA 2007 methodology for the development of clinical data standards: a report of the American College of Cardiology/American Heart Association Task Force on Clinical Data Standards. *Circulation,* 2007. 115(7): p. 936-43.
[71] Mehran, R., et al., Impact of bleeding on mortality after percutaneous coronary intervention results from a patient-level pooled analysis of the REPLACE-2 (randomized evaluation of PCI linking angiomax to reduced clinical events), ACUITY (acute catheterization and urgent intervention triage strategy), and HORIZONS-AMI (harmonizing outcomes with revascularization and stents in acute myocardial infarction) trials. JACC. *Cardiovascular interventions,* 2011. 4(6): p. 654-64.
[72] Mehran, R., et al., Standardized bleeding definitions for cardiovascular clinical trials: a consensus report from the Bleeding Academic Research Consortium. *Circulation*, 2011. 123(23): p. 2736-47.
[73] Brindis, R.G., et al., The American College of Cardiology-National Cardiovascular Data Registry (ACC-NCDR): building a national clinical data repository. *Journal of the American College of Cardiology*, 2001. 37(8): p. 2240-5.
[74] LaBresh, K.A., et al., Get with the guidelines for cardiovascular secondary prevention: pilot results. *Archives of internal medicine*, 2004. 164(2): p. 203-9.
[75] Peterson, E.D., et al., The NCDR ACTION Registry-GWTG: transforming contemporary acute myocardial infarction clinical care. *Heart,* 2010. 96(22): p. 1798-802.
[76] Chan, P.S., et al., Cardiac performance measure compliance in outpatients: the American College of Cardiology and National Cardiovascular Data Registry's PINNACLE (Practice Innovation And Clinical Excellence) program. *Journal of the American College of Cardiology,* 2010. 56(1): p. 8-14.
[77] Weintraub, W.S., et al., Comparative effectiveness of revascularization strategies. *The New England Journal of medicine*, 2012. 366(16): p. 1467-76.
[78] Brennan, J.M., et al., Linking the National Cardiovascular Data Registry CathPCI Registry with Medicare claims data: validation of a longitudinal cohort of elderly patients undergoing cardiac catheterization. Circulation. *Cardiovascular quality and outcomes*, 2012. 5(1): p. 134-40.
[79] Weintraub, W.S., et al., Prediction of long-term mortality after percutaneous coronary intervention in older adults: results from the National Cardiovascular Data Registry. *Circulation,* 2012. 125(12): p. 1501-10.
[80] Zwolak, R.M., Reimbursement for carotid stenting: unique challenges for medical centers and physicians. *Seminars in vascular surgery*, 2006. 19(2): p. 87-91.

[81] Holmes, D.R., Jr., et al., 2012 ACCF/AATS/SCAI/STS expert consensus document on transcatheter aortic valve replacement. *Journal of the American College of Cardiology*, 2012. 59(13): p. 1200-54.
[82] Bradley, E.H., et al., National efforts to improve door-to-balloon time results from the Door-to-Balloon Alliance. *Journal of the American College of Cardiology*, 2009. 54(25): p. 2423-9.
[83] Nestler, D.M., et al., Sustaining improvement in door-to-balloon time over 4 years: the Mayo clinic ST-elevation myocardial infarction protocol. Circulation. *Cardiovascular quality and outcomes*, 2009. 2(5): p. 508-13.
[84] Frieden, T.R. and D.M. Berwick, The "Million Hearts" initiative--preventing heart attacks and strokes. *The New England Journal of Medicine,* 2011. 365(13): p. e27.
[85] Million hearts: strategies to reduce the prevalence of leading cardiovascular disease risk factors--United States, 2011. MMWR. *Morbidity and mortality weekly report*, 2011. 60(36): p. 1248-51.
[86] Berwick, D.M., What 'patient-centered' should mean: confessions of an extremist. *Health affairs,* 2009. 28(4): p. w555-65.
[87] Reuben, D.B. and M.E. Tinetti, Goal-oriented patient care--an alternative health outcomes paradigm. *The New England Journal of Medicine,* 2012. 366(9): p. 777-9.
[88] Brindis, R. and J.A. Spertus, President's page: employing shared decision-making models to improve care and patient value: a cardiovascular professional initiative. *Journal of the American College of Cardiology,* 2010. 56(24): p. 2046-8.
[89] Mehran, R., et al., A simple risk score for prediction of contrast-induced nephropathy after percutaneous coronary intervention: development and initial validation. *Journal of the American College of Cardiology*, 2004. 44(7): p. 1393-9.
[90] Dangas, G.D., et al., Frequency and predictors of stent thrombosis after percutaneous coronary intervention in acute myocardial infarction. *Circulation*, 2011. 123(16): p. 1745-56.
[91] Stacey, D., et al., Decision aids for people facing health treatment or screening decisions. *Cochrane database of systematic reviews*, 2011(10): p. CD001431.
[92] Barry, M.J. and S. Edgman-Levitan, Shared decision making--pinnacle of patient-centered care. *The New England Journal of Medicine,* 2012. 366(9): p. 780-1.
[93] Barry, M.J., Shared decision making: informing and involving patients to do the right thing in health care. *The Journal of ambulatory care management,* 2012. 35(2): p. 90-8.
[94] Amsterdam, E.A., et al., Testing of low-risk patients presenting to the emergency department with chest pain: a scientific statement from the American Heart Association. *Circulation,* 2010. 122(17): p. 1756-76.
[95] Hess, E.P., et al., The chest pain choice decision aid: a randomized trial. Circulation. *Cardiovascular quality and outcomes*, 2012. 5(3): p. 251-9.
[96] Allen, L.A., et al., Decision Making in Advanced Heart Failure: A Scientific Statement From the American Heart Association. *Circulation,* 2012. 125(15): p. 1928-1952.
[97] Selby, J.V., A.C. Beal, and L. Frank, The Patient-Centered Outcomes Research Institute (PCORI) national priorities for research and initial research agenda. *JAMA: the Journal of the American Medical Association,* 2012. 307(15): p. 1583-4.
[98] Methodology Committee of the Patient-Centered Outcomes Research, I., Methodological standards and patient-centeredness in comparative effectiveness research: the PCORI perspective. *JAMA: the Journal of the American Medical Association,* 2012. 307(15): p. 1636-40.

[99] Berwick, D.M., Launching accountable care organizations--the proposed rule for the Medicare Shared Savings Program. *The New England Journal of medicine,* 2011. 364(16): p. e32.
[100] Blumenthal, D., Performance Improvement in Health Care - Seizing the Moment. *The New England Journal of Medicine*, 2012.
[101] Schoen, C., et al., New 2011 survey of patients with complex care needs in eleven countries finds that care is often poorly coordinated. *Health affairs,* 2011. 30(12): p. 2437-48.

In: Quality Improvement
Editors: K. W. Lobdell and S. C. Stamou
ISBN: 978-1-62417-390-5

Chapter 6

Appropriate Use of Medical Imaging

Thomas V. Johnson *
Sanger Heart and Vascular Institute, Charlotte, NC, US

Abstract

Medical imaging is a significant component in the medical landscape. Appropriate use of medical imaging constitutes a growing area of interest as a part of a national pursuit towards optimizing the quality of healthcare delivery. There are several ways that appropriate use can have a favorable impact on quality of care including cost efficiency, reduced rates of patient radiation exposure, and impact on accuracy of testing. Guidelines outlining appropriate use of imaging have been published, however, adoption into clinical practice has been incomplete. Understanding the reasons for this is an important first step in beginning the process of improving compliance with the guidelines. A multifaceted approach to enhance appropriate use of medical imaging is outlined in this chapter.

Introduction

Imaging is a critical part of the practice of medicine in the modern era. Choosing which procedure and when to use it is an important decision that has significant impact on the healthcare delivery in this country. There are multiple guidelines that define appropriate use, however, the translation of these guidelines into clinical practice has been poor. Quality improvement initiatives designed to improve compliance with recognized guidelines for appropriate use of medical imaging are emerging as an important part of the medical landscape.

Importance of Appropriate Use in Medical Imaging

There are several reasons why appropriate use of medical imaging is important. From the perspective of the national healthcare delivery system cost of unnecessary imaging is a factor.

* E-mail: TJohnson@carolinashealthcare.org.

Beyond this there are issues surrounding the quality of healthcare. Patient radiation exposure, diagnostic accuracy, potential adverse reactions to contrast with imaging, and incomplete diagnostic information for patient care are all potential concerns with inappropriate use of imaging procedures.

Medical imaging accounts for a significant percentage of the healthcare expenditures in this country. In 2008 Medicare part B spending on imaging was $14.1 billion dollars [1]. In the GAO report to Congress that outlined Medicare spending it was estimated that 20-30% of all medical imaging was done for unnecessary reasons. Reductions in reimbursement are already in place, but there are growing fears that while curbing costs these may unintentionally be adversely affecting access. A strategy to reduce unnecessary imaging is becoming an integral part in the fight to contain costs. Pre-approval for procedures and radiation benefits managers are already becoming common. These solutions are imperfect and have lead to increased inefficiencies in the system with additional beurocracy. The best solutions rely on the appropriate application of clinical guidelines to individual patients by their providers.

With the evolving technologies and the explosion in use of diagnostic imaging procedures there is a growing concern about the long-term risks from radiation exposure to patients. The number of CT scans performed in the United States has increased from 3 million in 1980 to 70 million per year. The increase in cardiovascular imaging was even greater outpacing the rise in use of non-cardiac advanced imaging procedures [2] (see figure 1). Many of these diagnostic-imaging procedures are associated with ionizing radiation. The biological effects from ionizing radiation include the formation of hydroxyl radicals from the interaction of x-rays and water molecules, which can lead to damage in cellular DNA. The resulting point mutations, chromosomal translocations and gene fusions can all lead to increased risk of cancer [3]. The estimates of linear risk from exposure to low levels of radiation is mostly based on the study of survivors from the atomic blast in Japan and is reported in the BIER VII report [4]. Analysis of this data has shown a direct correlation between the level of radiation exposure and risk of cancer. When estimating these risks it is important to remember radiation exposure is cumulative across the patients lifetime, so not only is the amount of radiation exposure related to the type of testing, but also to the number of times the patient may have that test over the coarse of their lifetime. When analyzing exposure this is typically expressed in terms of the effective biological absorption of ionizing radiation per unit of mass in the patient.

Furthermore, based on the focused nature of diagnostic imaging radiation typically effects one or two organ systems. For example, with a head CT the brain receives the highest level of radiation whereas the radiation exposure to the lung or stomach is considerably less. For these reasons radiation exposure from various procedures is usually reported in grays (Gy) (1 Gy = 1 joule/kg) or milligrays (mGy) as a relative organ dose.

Typical estimates of exposure from various procedures are outlined in Table 1. Extrapolating the data from the BIER report estimates of cancer risk and the data on procedure specific radiation exposure one can then get a numeric estimate of the relative risk of various diagnostic imaging tests (see Table 2).

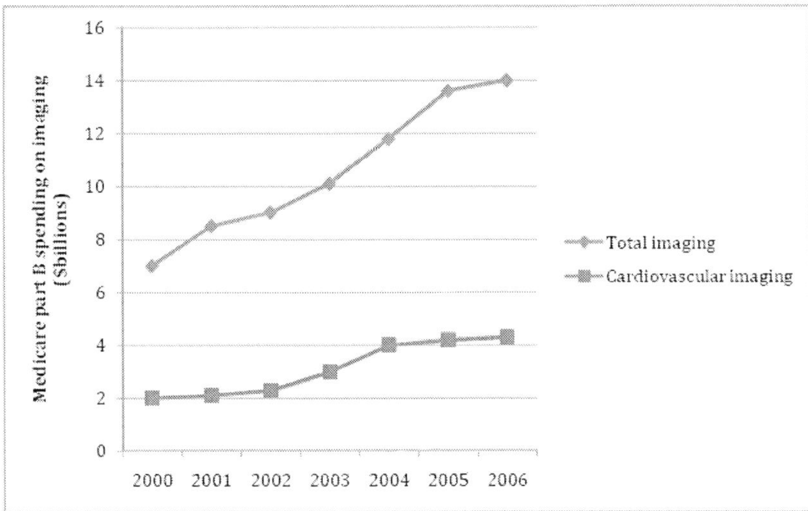

Adapted from : Shaw LJ, et al. *J. Am. Coll. Cardiol. Imag*. 2010; 3: 789-784.

Figure 1. Medicare outpatient spending on diagnostic imaging and cardiovascular imaging over a 6 year period.

Table 1. Radiation Exposure of Various Radiological Procedures

Study Type	Relative Organ	Radiation exposure mGy
PA and lateral chest x ray	Lung	.01
Adult Abdominal CT	Stomach	10
Adult Head CT	Brain	95
Myocardial Perfusion imaging (Tc 99)	Lung	5
Myocardial Perfusion imaging (Thallium 207)	Lung	12

Table 2. Relative risk of cancer based on imaging procedure

Procedure	Radiation exposure	Risk of cancer
Chest x-ray	0.1 mSv	1:100,000
CT Chest	8 mSv	1:3000
64 Slice CT heart	13 mSv	1:1000
Thallium stress test	25 mSv	1:750
PET scan	32 mSv	1:650

Based on these risk estimates approximately 29,000 cases of future cancers will develop from the radiation exposure due to CT scans performed in 2007 alone. [5] The most effective way of decreasing the medical populations exposure to radiation from diagnostic imaging is to reduce the number of studies being performed. [6] Since up to 30% of studies are deemed inappropriate, application of appropriate use guidelines into clinical practice can substantially reduce the number of imaging procedures performed without having a negative impact on the individual patients care.

Diagnostic accuracy of testing is not often considered when it comes to appropriate use, however, it can be adversely affected by inappropriate imaging. The diagnostic accuracy of any imaging as defined by the predictive positive and negative values for the test is determined by three factors: 1) the sensitivity of the test for the disease being tested, 2) the specificity of the test for the disease being tested and, 3) the prevalence of the disease in the patient population being tested.

The first two of these are determined by the receiver operating characteristics of the imaging procedure itself. The last, however, can be affected by the choice of patients being sent for imaging. The guidelines for appropriate use are based in part on the estimation of pretest probability for any given patient of having the disease in question. In certain clinical scenarios there are markers of risk that help define this probability. In patients with low risk of having the disease the yield of diagnostic imaging will be low. Based on a careful assessment of the disease specific risk to the patient diagnostic imaging is often classified as inappropriate for patients at low risk of having the disease. Testing of those patients classified as inappropriate based on low pretest probability creates a low prevalence of disease and leads to a higher rate of false positive imaging. For example for stress cardiac thallium imaging studies sensitivity is 90% and specificity is 75%. If patients with a low pretest probability are being tested (prevalence < 5%) this will result in 24 false positive exams for every 100 patients. The higher rate of false positive imaging will obviously have adverse impact on patient care resulting in misdiagnosis, overtreatment and often further unnecessary testing with resultant risks of complications.

The risk of adverse reactions with contrast agents used in many imaging exams should also be considered. Reactions range from mild flushing and rash to nephrotoxicity and severe anaphylactic reactions. The total incidence of reactions with high osmolality ionic contrast agents is estimated at 5-15% [7]. With lower osmolality ionic agents the incidence is lower with incidences between 0.2% - 0.7% [8, 9]. Fortunately severe reactions have a much lower risk with an estimated incidence of 0.1-0.2% for high osmolality agents and 0.01-0.02% for low osmoality agents [10]. Although the risks are relatively low on an individual patient basis the population based risk for patients undergoing unnecessary imaging is actually high.

Finally, there are the imaging procedures that are not performed which based on standard of care should have been performed. Quality of care centered on evidence-based medicine guides the clinician in determining when and what type of testing should be performed.

When tests are not done when indicated this can have a significant negative impact on patient care. An appropriate diagnosis may be missed leading to delayed or incorrect treatment of patients. The incidence of this is more difficult to estimate than statistics for inappropriate testing, however it seems likely this is not inconsequential.

Appropriate Use Guidelines for Medical Imaging

Quality of care in medical imaging is often difficult to quantify. Although there are number of evidence based guidelines for various prevention and treatment algorithms, there are very limited prospective clinical trials or evidence based studies that can be used to quantify quality in medical imaging. Because of this outcomes measures for assessing quality are difficult to apply. Instead we can apply surrogate markers for quality in medical imaging such as those proposed by the Duke University Think Tank on Cardiovascular Imaging (see Table 3) [11]. One of these markers is patient selection. Patient selection is based on " doing the right test at the right time on the right patient".

Table 3. Surrogate markers for assessing quality of imaging

Quality markers
Patient selection
Image acquisition
Image interpretation
Results communication

Adapted from Douglass P, et al. *J. Am. Coll. Cardiol.* 2006; 48: 2141- 2151.

Appropriate use of medical imaging is all about patient selection. This is why we choose appropriate use as a quality metric for medical imaging. The definitions for appropriate use have been developed by various professional medical societies based on expert consensus and literature review. These have been compiled, updated, and published in the form of clinical guidelines for radiology in the ACR Appropriateness Criteria [12] and for cardiac imaging in the Appropriateness criteria for echocardiography [13], the Appropriateness criteria for cardiac radionuclide imaging [14], the Appropriateness criteria for cardiac CT [15], and the Appropriateness criteria for diagnostic cardiac catheterization [16].

These documents were designed to help clinicians identify clinical scenarios where imaging can provide a positive impact on patient care. The guidelines are organized into clinical scenarios, which are categorized as "appropriate," "inappropriate," or "uncertain." Appropriate indications are those in which there is general agreement imaging would be indicated. Inappropriate indications are those in which there is general agreement imaging would not be beneficial.

Finally, uncertain indications are those for which there may be some benefit but there is lack of consensus among experts because of incomplete or inconclusive support in the literature. Although no set of guidelines can cover all possible clinical scenarios the appropriate use criteria for imaging do cover the vast majority of indications for which testing is done in clinical practice. Several studies have shown that 90-93% of imaging tests ordered in clinical practice could be classified based on the appropriate use criteria [17, 18].

The application of the appropriate use criteria into clinical practice has been disappointing. Utilizing the criteria in the imaging guidelines 15-20% of imaging procedures were classified as inappropriate [19, 20]. In a survey of physicians only 2.4% reported that they utilized the ACR Appropriateness criteria for decision making when ordering imaging [21]. These figures provide evidence of a significant gap in the application of evidence-based utilization of medical imaging in the current delivery of healthcare.

Quality Improvement Process for Appropriate Use

While practice guidelines are instrumental in defining appropriate use they are just one component in an effective quality improvement initiative. As outlined previously publication of guidelines on appropriate use of medical imaging have not translated well into clinical practice. Development and publication of clinical guidelines by themselves are weak tools for implementing change at the clinical level [22, 23, 24]. Moving knowledge from research and guidelines to direct patient care at the community level remains a significant challenge.

There are multiple examples of the lag between the establishment of evidence-based therapies with positive impact on patient care and their promulgation to the vast majority of patients. Beta-blockers for the treatment of acute myocardial infarction 15 years after the publication of the Beta-blocker Heart Attack trial were still only prescribed for 62.5% of patients [25]. Despite the publication of treatment guidelines recommending the demonstrated benefit for early reperfusion of acute myocardial infarction in 1996 [26] six years later in 2002 nearly one third of eligible patients still did not receive percutaneous intervention or fibrinolytic therapy [27]. For meaningful improvement it is necessary to identify the barriers to implementation of clinical knowledge into clinical practice.

There are several common problems associated with implementation of clinical guidelines. These include but are not limited to reliance on passive diffusion of knowledge, resistance to perceived physician autonomy, concerns regarding clinical efficiency, disagreement with guideline content, practice characteristics, incentives, regulations, and patient factors. [28, 29]. The publication of clinical guidelines in scientific journals has long been the traditional method of clinician education done on a national scale. Despite this and the increased utilization of non-traditional sources for dissemination such as web-based sites the clinician's awareness of clinical guidelines remains poor. In a study of pediatricians it was found that only 50% were aware of the guidelines for treatment of otitis media [30]. Beyond this there is also variance between the clinicians perceived compliance with guidelines and the actual compliance with a significant degree of overestimation by clinicians [31]. Together these create a significant gap in the effective dissemination of knowledge to the practicing clinician.

Another potential roadblock to implementation at the clinician level is the degree to which clinicians feel their clinical efficiency may be negatively impacted with attempts at incorporation of guidelines which are often complex. Attempts at utilization of computer prompts for clinically relevant recommendations have met with only mixed success in large part due to inefficient intrusions in the daily work flow [32]. In addition clinicians may disagree with guideline content or perceive an encroachment on their autonomy. This has been explored by researchers who find compliance may be related to the guidelines compatibility with existing beliefs, complexity, costs, "observability" and "trialability" [33]. Guidelines that were uncomplicated, consistent with previous clinical idioms, and could easily be tried and observed by clinicians were more frequently adopted into clinical practice [34]. This may be particularly relevant to guidelines on appropriate use of medical imaging which are complex with limited observability for the practicing physician. Finally, without a readily accessible reference and the number of clinical scenarios numbering in the hundreds it is difficult for practicing clinicians to have a working knowledge of the recommendations that can be efficiently applied in the typical practice setting.

Practice setting and clinician demographics need to be considered when identifying barriers to implementation. Barriers that exist in smaller "private practice" settings may not apply to larger system based provider organizations. For example, smaller groups may not have the resources to dedicate to an ongoing quality improvement protocol to assure adherence with guidelines, but instead rely on the individual clinician to maintain proficiency. This is particularly germane in the practice of appropriate use for clinical imaging where the ordering clinician may not be a part of the organization providing the services ordered. Oversight of ordering patterns becomes a burden on the provider of imaging with limited control over the multiple referring clinicians. Secondly there is a difference in compliance between academic and community based settings as well as outpatient versus hospital settings

[35]. Clinician demographics can have similar differential effects on compliance. Age plays a role with older physicians being less likely to adopt and practice clinical guidelines [36]. Furthermore, practice specialty also has an impact on compliance with imaging guidelines. Specialists have a higher rate of appropriate use of medical imaging than primary care physicians.

Finally patient factors can play a role in affecting appropriate use of medical imaging. Patients often have a preconceived notion that diagnostic imaging is associated with quality of medical care. Although medical imaging may not be clinically appropriate patients perceive the absence of testing as incomplete care pressuring physicians to perform more testing to maintain patient satisfaction.

Regulatory efforts that are currently employed or are being instituted to curb inappropriate use of medical imaging are nationally based initiatives that fail to address the barriers noted above. Requirements for appropriate use tracking as a part of the standards for lab accreditation are the first steps in this initiative. The subsequent step will be to add the requirement that appropriate use be maintained above a certain level for imaging labs to remain accredited and thus receive reimbursement for procedures. Unfortunately this does not specify how imaging labs can accomplish this leaving the burden for designing and implementing a quality improvement initiative on the individual lab.

Recognizing this the efforts at reducing inappropriate imaging will likely come from the providers of medical imaging. To accomplish this will require the application of principles from translational medicine. The science of translational medicine and quality improvement is young but several key principles are emerging. First, at its core this is about changing individual clinician behavior. To do this efforts must incorporate an understanding of the process that occurs with conversion of knowledge into clinical practice. There are three stages involved in translation of medical guidelines into medical practice: awareness, acknowledgement, and adoption [37]. From awareness and acknowledgement to adoption the clinician goes through three cognitive phases: 1) the declarative phase, 2) the procedural phase, and 3) the autonomous phase [38, 39]. In the declarative phase knowledge is incorporated into the clinicians awareness. This is typically where traditional didactic lectures and journal articles have impact. The clinician actively evaluates the data and incorporates that data into their knowledge base. For example, the clinician recognizes and accepts the impact of beta-blockers on certain patients with heart failure. It is not until the second phase or procedural phase that the clinician actually attempts to integrate this knowledge into practice. Here the clinician will develop rules for incorporation of that knowledge into the daily practice. To take our example the clinician will actively create a set of rules defining heart failure and which patients to think about utilization of beta-blockers. In the final phase these rules become automatic and do not require any special efforts at recall on the part of the clinician. It is in this final stage of adoption that the knowledge will increase the clinician's efficiency in clinical practice. For this reason it is important to complete all three phases of cognitive learning which leads to positive reinforcement. Awareness and acknowledgement as we have said before is acquired based on traditional methods such as guideline dissemination and continuing medical education and has generally been the focus of most efforts. Despite longstanding efforts knowledge dissemination remains imperfect. Furthermore, adoption is even more complex with limited data to guide us. Accepting this framework is an important step in developing meaningful efforts for affecting positive change in clinicians ordering patterns [40]. A multifaceted strategy encompassing provider education, reminder and support systems, audit and feedback, patient education, and regulations is the best method for accomplishing this goal [41]. This strategy has been employed with success in a similar quality initiative to affect clinician performance in imaging interpretation [42]. We will explore how this type of a program can be applied to the problem of inappropriate use of medical imaging.

Clinician education regarding appropriate use of medical imaging should not rely solely on dissemination of guidelines and continuing medical education. Traditional didactic lectures and journal articles don't contextualize the information into the practice setting where the clinician is actually seeing the patient. A more focused program with case based examples and teaching is more effective in achieving the goal of more appropriate ordering patterns. Combining traditional lectures with case presentations and audience participation enhances the transition from declarative knowledge (stage 1) to procedural knowledge (stage 2). This helps the clinician connect the knowledge with a series of rules that can be applied to everyday clinical scenarios. Furthermore, educational programs should be focused on demonstrated areas of non-compliance. Some patterns of use and inappropriate use are recognized at the national level. For example, with cardiovascular imaging inappropriate imaging in patients with chest pain and low clinical risk and as part of a preoperative evaluation constitute the two most common areas of inappropriate use in numerous studies on appropriate use applications in clinical practice [18, 43, 44].

At the same time there can be variations in usage patterns based on region, practice setting and provider type [20]. For this reason it is important to individualize ordering patterns based on the lab itself and the providers utilizing the imaging lab. This type of information can be gleaned from an initial survey of cases to assess compliance with guidelines at baseline. A random group of consecutive cases from the imaging lab is reviewed to assess the indication for testing as ordered by the providers. These testing indications can then be categorized as appropriate, inappropriate, uncertain, or unclassified according to the guidelines. The first three categories are found delineated in the guidelines themselves. Indications not specifically addressed in the guidelines are identified as unclassified. From this data one can then do a statistical analysis to determine the frequency of ordering indications for the lab. More specifically the most common inappropriate ordering practices can be recognized. This presents a target of opportunity to tailor an educational profile to address the most common errors. For example in a cardiovascular imaging lab with typical patterns of usage the education would focus on how to identify patients cardiovascular risk to avoid ordering testing in low risk patients and how to identify preoperative cardiac risk to guide test ordering. A typical program might consist of a succinct review of the determinants of cardiac risk in chest pain patients along with the components of the cardiovascular preoperative evaluation followed by a series of hypothetical patient scenarios in which the clinician must decide which if any testing would be appropriate.

A second component of an initiative for improvement involves system support and tools. Guidelines for medical imaging are lengthy and complex as stated earlier. The busy practicing clinician needs easily referenced documents or non-obtrusive reminders to help with the multiple clinical decisions regarding imaging orders that are encountered on a daily basis. The American Heart Association recognizes the importance of this and is working to develop order templates to encourage more complete translation of evidence statements into clinical practice [8]. Specifically designed order forms can be an effective reminder to clinicians at the point of care. A well-organized form with the appropriate indications grouped by category can prompt the clinician when ordering an imaging test. If the indication for which the test is being ordered is not on the order form it alerts the physician that this may not be an appropriate use.

In addition precise parameters such as frequency of testing and appropriate time intervals for follow up may be included on the order form. Single page order forms for cardiovascular stress imaging, echocardiography, CT scanning, MRI, etc. can be designed to meet these criteria (see Figure 4 for sample forms). In addition these forms can include algorithms and risk assessment tools that can be applied by the clinician at the point of care to determine eligibility for further imaging. Specific information that addresses concern areas identified in the baseline survey are often helpful. For example with cardiovascular stress imaging we recognized 2 common problems: 1) correctly identifying cardiac risk in patients with chest pain and 2) correctly identifying preoperative risk to guide ordering further testing. On the reverse side of the order form the definitions and tools for calculating cardiac risk in patients with chest pain and as part of the preoperative evaluation are listed (see figure 4). With the rapid increase in utilization of computer order entry as part of a comprehensive electronic medical record these types of interventions and support will be made easier. Algorithms to assist clinicians in ordering testing appropriately can be embedded in the system guiding the clinician through the appropriate questions to determine indications for testing.

Audit and feedback form the third part of the quality improvement process. After institution of educational efforts and system support tools such as ordering forms it is important to provide feedback to clinicians. Individual review of performance benchmarked against peers can be a powerful tool for motivation and change. In addition providing feedback is an integral part in converting knowledge into the autonomous phase of cognitive learning. Identifying areas of persistent errors forms a negative feedback loop that allows the clinician to adjust and correct image ordering patterns favorably. After completion of formal training clinicians receive very little oversight. Incorporating new knowledge into practice is often done in a vacuum with very little guidance. Errors in application may not be apparent to the practitioner. Because of this feedback provides the clinician with supervision that leads to more accurate application of the rules and the confidence to allow the process to become more automatic. This is even more apparent when appropriate use ordering is done in the electronic environment where systems can be designed for immediate feedback. Ordering CT angiography of the chest to rule out pulmonary embolus for example might require calculation of the pre test probability of pulmonary embolus based on Well's criteria. This would be done on a sub menu of the order screen for CT angiography for suspected pulmonary embolus. If the probability is calculated as low the clinician would receive instant prompting that the test is likely inappropriate. Over a short time interval these patterns for image ordering become second nature enhancing the confidence of the clinician and increasing the efficiency of the practice.

Patient education will be necessary to avoid "doctor shopping" and poor patient satisfaction. Patient expectations can create a pressure on clinicians to overuse medical imaging. Educating patients to the risks of medical imaging (radiation exposure, false positive imaging, etc.) will help patients to understand that imaging procedures are not to be taken lightly. In cases of inappropriate use the potential benefits are outweighed by these risks. Patient education begins with the clinician at the point of care. A careful discussion by the clinician with the patient highlighting the decision making process surrounding an imaging test can alleviate patient concerns regarding the quality of their medical care. The clinician, who has incorporated the knowledge, has the system support tools and the confidence from a feedback program will be well prepared to have this type of interaction with positive impact.

Despite all of these efforts there will likely be some persistent outliers who continue to have high rates of inappropriate usage. For these cases regulations will be necessary. As stated earlier accreditation organizations have recognized the value of tracking appropriate use. As part of the accreditation process for echocardiography and cardiac nuclear perfusion laboratories must submit data on test indications and appropriate use rates based on current guidelines. Currently this data is based on self-review and is not corroborated by the accrediting body. In the future this data will need to be be validated. For example, the lab will have to submit 30 consecutive studies from any given dates along with hospital or office notes from the clinician outlining the indications for test ordering for each study. Based on this a realistic estimate of appropriate use rates can be made. Accreditation can then be denied to imaging centers with persistently high rates of inappropriate usage.

Tying reimbursement rates with accreditation creates a new model for value-based compensation as opposed to volume-based compensation. Motivated by these incentives imaging centers will then be responsible for tracking the outliers who are non compliant with appropriate use guidelines. If they are unresponsive to quality initiatives for improvement their privileges for test ordering in the imaging center can be revoked. While undesirable these types of interventions may be necessary to obtaining optimal outcomes.

CONCLUSION

Appropriate use of medical imaging will be one of the important components of healthcare delivery in the future of value-based medicine which emphasizes quality and cost efficiency. Potential cost savings from reduction in unnecessary imaging could have a significant impact on reducing healthcare expenditures without a negative impact on patient care. Furthermore, reductions in rates of inappropriate imaging will reduce patient radiation exposure from medical imaging providing a substantial impact on decreasing risks for development of radiation induced cancer. Finally, appropriate use of imaging will improve the accuracy of diagnostic testing based on patient selection.

Guidelines for medical imaging have been published to help clinicians decide when medical imaging would be considered appropriate. Unfortunately compliance with recommendations from the guidelines has been relatively poor with an estimated 15-30% of all imaging deemed to be inappropriate. Multiple barriers to implementation of guidelines have been identified including reliance on clinician initiated self education, complexity of appropriate use criteria, negative impact on clinician efficiency, and patients preconceived ideas correlating quality of care with diagnostic testing.

A systematic multifaceted approach to quality improvement is necessary to have a favorable impact on appropriate use of cardiac imaging. Focused clinician education combining traditional didactic programs with contextualized learning is the first step. Secondly, clinicians require support tools such as specifically designed ordering forms (or system prompts on electronic ordering systems) to help make the criteria for appropriateness accessible at the point of care. Feedback to individual clinicians with peer review is another important component that leads to improved compliance with guidelines. Finally regulations for imaging centers regarding rates of appropriate utilization may be necessary from a national perspective to achieve the goal of effectively reducing inappropriate imaging.

REFERENCES

[1] GAO Medicare Part B Imaging Services. *Rapid Spending Growth and Shift to Physician Offices Indicate Need for CMS to Consider Additional Management Practices.* http://www.gao.gov/new.items/d08452.pdf 2010 Accessed November 11, 2009.

[2] Department of Health and Human Services: Office of Inspector General Growth in Advanced Imaging Paid Under the Medicare Physician Fee Schedule http://oig.hhs.gov/oei/reports/oei-01-06-00260.pdf 2010 Accessed November 10, 2009.

[3] Mitelman F, Johansson B, Mertens FE. Mitelman database of chromosome aberrations in cancer. *Cancer Genome Anatomy Project,* 2007.

[4] Bier VII Report. *Health Risks from Exposure to Low Levels of Ionizing Radiation.* June 2005.

[5] Berrington de Gonzales, A; Mahesh,M; Kim,K; Bhargavan,M; Lewis,R; Mettler,F, Land,C. Projected cancer risks from computed tomographic scans performed in the United States in 2007. *Arch. Intern. Med.* 2009; 169 (22): 2071-2077.

[6] Brener,D; Hall,E. Computed tomography- An increasing source of radiation exposure. *N. Engl. J. Med.* 2007; 357: 2277-2284.

[7] Dillman JR, Strouse PJ, Ellis JH, Cohan RH, Jan SC. Incidence and severity of acute allergic-like reactions to i.v. nonionic iodinated contrast material in children. *AJR Am. J. Roentgenol.* 2007; 188:1643–1647.

[8] Cochran ST, Bomyea K, Sayre JW. Trends in adverse events after IV administration of contrast media. *AJR Am. J. Roentgenol.* 2001; 176:1385–1388.

[9] Wang CL, Cohan RH, Ellis JH, Caoili EM, Wang G, Francis IR. Frequency, outcome, and appropriateness of treatment of nonionic iodinated contrast media reactions. *AJR Am. J. Roent- genol.* 2008; 191: 409–415.

[10] *ACR Manuel on contrast media.*

[11] Douglas P, Iskandrian AE, Krumholz HM. Achieving quality in cardiovascular imaging. Proceedings from the American College of Cardiology–Duke University Medical Center Think Tank on Quality in Cardiovascular Imaging. *J. Am. Coll. Cardiol.* 2006;48:2141-2151.

[12] *ACR Appropriate use criteria.*

[13] Douglas P, Garcia M, Haines D, Lai W, et al. ACCF/ASE/AHA/ASNC/ HFSA/HRS/SCAI/SCCM/SCCT/SCMR 2011 Appropriate Use Criteria for Echocardiography. *J. Am. Coll. Cardiol.,* 2011; 57: 1126-1166.

[14] Hendel R, Berman D, Heidenreich P, Pellikka P, et al. ACCF/ASNC/ACR/AHA/ASE/SCCT/SCMR/SNM 2009 Appropriate Use Criteria for Cardiac Radionuclide Imaging. *J. Am. Coll. Cardiol.,* 2009; 53: 2201-2229.

[15] Taylor A, Cerqueira M, Hodgson J, Mark D, et al. ACCF/SCCT/ACR/ AHA/ASE/ASNC/NASCI/SCAI/SCMR 2010 Appropriate Use Criteria for Cardiac Computed Tomography. *J. Am. Coll. Cardiol.* 2010, 56; 1864-1894.

[16] Patel M, Bailey S, Bonow R, Chan P, et al. ACCF/SCAI/AATS/AHA/ ASE/ASNC/HFSA/HRS/SCCM/SCCT/SCMR/STS 2012 Appropriate Use Criteria for Diagnostic Catheterization. *J. Am. Coll. Cardiol.* 2012, (published online May 2012).

[17] Aggarwal N, Punsak, W, Karon, B, Miller F, et al. Application of the Appropriateness Criteria for Echocardiography in an Academic Medical Center. *JASE.* 2010; 23: 267-274.

[18] Gibbons R, Miller T, Hodge D, et al. Application of Appropriateness Criteria to Stress Single-Photon Emission Computed Tomography Sestamibi Studies and Stress Echocardiograms in an Academic Medical Center. *J. Am. Coll. Cardiol.* 2008; 51: 1283-1289.
[19] Hendel R, Cerqueira M, Douglas P, et al. A Multicenter Assessment of the Use of Single-Photon Emission Computed Tomography Myocardial Perfusion Imaging With Appropriateness Criteria. *J. Am. Coll. Cardiol.* 2010; 55: 156-162.
[20] Willens H, Orlando G, Heldman A, et al. Adherence to Appropriateness Criteria for Transthoracic Echocardiography: Comparisons Between a Regional Department of Veterans Affairs Health Care System and Academic Practice and Between Physicians and Mid-Level Providers. *JASE.* 2009; 22:793-799.
[21] Bautista A, Burgos A, Nichol B, et al. Do Clinicians Use the American College of Radiology Appropriateness Criteria in the Management of Their Patients? *AJR.* 2009; 192: 1581-1585.
[22] Davis D.A., Thomson M.A., Oxman A.D. and Haynes R.B. Evidence for the effectiveness of CME: a review of 50 randomized controlled trials. *JAMA* 1992;268:1111-1117.
[23] Bero L.A., Grilli R. and Grimshaw J.M. et al. Closing the gap between research and practice: an overview of systematic reviews of interventions to promote the implementation of research findings. *BMJ* 1998; 317:465-468.
[24] Woolf SH and Atkins D. The evolving role of prevention in health care: Contributions of the U.S. Preventive Services Task Force. *Am. J. Prev. Med.* 2001;20(3S):13-2011.
[25] Stafford RS, Radley DC. The underutilization of cardiac medications of proven benefit, 1990 to 2002. *J. Am. Coll. Cardiol.* 2003; 41:56-61.
[26] Ryan TJ, Anderson JL, Antman EM, et al. ACC/AHA guidelines for the management of patients with acute myocardial infarction: executive summary: a report of the American College of Cardiology/American Heart Association Task Force on Practice Guide- lines (Committee on Management of Acute Myocardial Infarction). *Circulation* 1996; 94:2341-50.
[27] National Registry of Myocardial Infarction. NMRI 4 quarterly data report 2002. South San Francisco, Calif.: *Genentech.,* 2002.
[28] Cabana MD, Rand CS, Powe NR, Wu AW, Wilson MH, Abboud PC, et al. Why don't physicians follow clinical practice guidelines? A framework for improvement. *JAMA.* 1999;282:1458-1465.
[29] Davis D, Taylor-Vaisey A. Translating guidelines into practice A systematic review of theoretic concepts, practical experience and research evidence in the adoption of clinical practice guidelines. *Can. Med. Assoc. J.* 1997;157:408-16.
[30] Christakis D.A. and Rivara F.P. Pediatricians' awareness of and attitudes about four clinical practice guidelines. *Pediatrics* 1998;101:825-830.
[31] Michael A. Steinman, MD, Melissa A. Fischer, MD, Med, Michael G. Shlipak, MD, MPH, Hayden B. Bosworth, PhD, et al Clinician awareness of adherence to hypertension guidelines. *Am. J. Med.* 2004; 117: 747-754.
[32] Hunt DL, Haynes RB, Hanna SE, Smith K. Effects of computer-based clinical decision support systems on physician performance and patient outcomes: a systematic review. *JAMA* 1998; 280: 1339-1346.
[33] Rogers EM. Lessons for guidelines from the diffusion of innovations. Jt *Comm. J. Qual. Improv.* 1995;21:324-8.

[34] Grilli R, Lomas J. Evaluating the message: the relationship between compli- ance rate and the subject of a practice guideline. *Med. Care* 1994; 32:202-13.
[35] Ward P, Krauss D, Mansour, I, Lemiux N, et al. Comparison of the Clinical Application of the American College of Cardiology Foundation/American Society of Echocardiography Appropriateness Criteria for Outpatient Transthoracic Echocardiography in Academic and Community Practice Settings. *JASE* 2009:22 (12):1375-1381.
[36] Ferrier BM, Woodward CA, Cohen M, Williams AP. Clinical practice guide- lines. New-to-practice family physicians' attitudes. *Can. Fam. Physician* 1996; 42:463-8.
[37] Davis D, Taylor-Vaisey A. Translating guidelines into practice A systematic review of theoretic concepts, practical experience and research evidence in the adoption of clinical practice guidelines. *Can. Med. Assoc. J.* 1997;157:408-16.
[38] Fitts PM. Perceptual motor skill learning. In: Melton AW, ed. *Categories of human learning*. New York: Academic Press; 1964.
[39] Fitts PM, Posner MI. Human performance. Belmont (CA); 1967.
[40] Green L, Seifert C. Translation of Research Into Practice: Why We Can't "Just Do It". *JABFM* 2005; 18: 541-545.
[41] Shojania KG, McDonald KM, Watcher RM,. Closing the quality gap: a critical analysis of quality improvement strategies; Vol 2. *Technical Review* 9(Prepared by the Stanfor). Rockville, MD: Agency for Healthcare Research and Quality; 2004 Sep. AHRQ Publication No. 04-0051-2. 32.
[42] Johnson T, Symanski J, Patel S, Rose G. Improvement in the Assessment of Diastolic Function in a Clinical Echocardiography Laboratory Following Implementation of a Quality Improvement Initiative. *JASE* 2011; 24: 1169-1179.
[43] McCully R, Pellikka P, Hodge D, Araoz P, et al. Applicability of Appropriateness Criteria for Stress ImagingSimilarities and Differences Between Stress Echocardiography and Single-Photon Emission Computed Tomography Myocardial Perfusion Imaging Criteria. *Circulation: Cardiovascular Imaging*, 2009; 2: 213-218.
[44] Ward, Krauss D, Mansour I, Lemieux N, et al. Comparison of the Clinical Application of the American College of Cardiology Foundation/American Society of Echocardiography Appropriateness Criteria for Outpatient Transthoracic Echocardiography in Academic and Community Practice Settings. *JASE*, 2009; 22:1375-1381.

SECTION FIVE: CARDIOVASCULAR SURGERY

In: Quality Improvement
Editors: K. W. Lobdell and S. C. Stamou
ISBN: 978-1-62417-390-5

Chapter 7

QUALITY IMPROVEMENT AND SURGICAL CHECKLISTS

Antonio D. Lassaletta, Nassrene Y. Elmadhun and Frank W. Sellke*

Division of Cardiothoracic Surgery,
Cardiovascular Research Center,
Warren Alpert Medical School of Brown University, Providence, RI, US

ABSTRACT

Sweeping changes in the culture of safety in perioperative care have occurred over the past decade. This has in part been sparked by the realization that half of all surgical complications, whether minor or major, have been deemed as preventable. Checklist use had revolutionized safety protocols in other sectors such as manufacturing and the airline industry. Thus, in 2008 when the World Health Organization released a simple yet universal safety checklist protocol to be used world-wide, many hospitals quickly embraced the new pathway. Despite a hugely successful pilot study of 8 hospitals across the globe, several follow-up studies question whether these marked improvements were due to the effectiveness of the checklist itself, or concomitant cultural changes which occurred with its implementation. Regardless, it's clear that improvements are occurring, though further investigation into causality are desperately needed as implementation of surgical safety protocols are becoming ubiquitous in both the industrialized and developing world.

INTRODUCTION

By 2008, it was estimated thatthere were 234 millionsurgical procedures each year worldwide. [1] With the rate of major surgical complications in developed countries ranging from 3% to 16% and half of these complications being deemed as preventable, [2-4] one

* Corresponding Author: Frank W. Sellke, MD - Division of Cardiothoracic Surgery, Cardiovascular Research Center, Warren Alpert Medical School of Brown University, 2 Dudley Street, MOC 360, Providence, RI 02905. E-mail: fsellke@lifespan.org. Ph: (401) 444-2732. Fax: (401) 444-2380.

could estimate upwards of 37 million preventable surgical complications annually. In this same time frame, the death rate for major surgery in industrialized countries was estimated at 0.4 to 0.8% and in developing countries an astonishing 5% to 10%. In the developing world, this was partly attributed to the mortality rate of general anesthesia alone, which was reported to be as high as 1 in 150 in parts of sub-Saharan Africa. [2]

With the business world focused on a quality standard of six sigma (six standard deviations), or only 3.4 defects per million produced, the medical world was lagging far behind. Confronted with strong evidence of significant public heath harm secondary to inadequate patient safety, the World Health Organization (WHO) held an international consortium in 2007 to clearly identify problems and derive a systematic approach toreduce surgical morbidity and mortality.

CREATIONOF THE WHO SURGICAL CHECKLIST

The need for safer surgical practices was clear. With nearly 1 in 25 people in the world undergoing surgery each yearfor an extremely wide range of indications ranging from emergent life-saving procedures to elective cosmetic operations, identifying where errors occur, what type of errors occur, and why these errors occur was no simple task. Furthermore, creating a universal protocol that was concise yet applicable to thousands of different procedures was equally as daunting.

The problem as defined by the WHO was that "complications of surgical care have become a major cause of death and disability worldwide." [2] Thus, the WHO applied a systematic approach to addressing the problem by identifying and addressing four underlying challenges to improving surgical safety and successfully measuring outcomes. The first challenge was validating the problem as a real and significant public health concern. While the WHO had previously placed a large emphasis on providing essential surgical care in areas of high need and low access, [5] the parallel need to improve surgical safety did not receive as much recognition. [2] The second challenge was to improve data collection and reporting of surgical outcomes globally, as there existed a wide variation in the collection of consistent quality data of surgical volume, morbidity, mortality, and outcomes. The third challenge involved addressing the inconsistencies in existing good safety practices such as the appropriate and timely administration of perioperative antibiotics, which even in rich countries was administered erratically, or the safe administration of general anesthesia which varied wildly in developing countries. [2] The fourth and final challenge dealt with the intrinsic complexity of surgery and the delivery of surgical healthcare. A surgical procedure alone consists of dozens of critical steps, and management of perioperative care involves anarray of complex steps beginning with the identification of the correct patient and procedure to ensuring a correct instrument count at the end of the case. [2]

With the contribution of nearly 100 international experts, in 2008 the WHO released the *Safe Surgery Saves Lives* checklist with 19 items aimed at preventing perioperative errors. [2] This universal protocol was designed to be a simple set of surgical safety standards organized as a checklist to be used in the operating room. The checklist was divided into three parts: the 'Sign In' before the induction of anesthesia, the 'Time Out' before the skin incision, and the 'Sign Out' before the patient leaves the operating room. The 'Sign In' confirms patient identity, correct site, correct surgical procedure, and that consent has been obtained. An anesthesia safety check is also to be performed at this time which includes monitoring oxygenation with a pulse oximeter. The 'Sign In' also reviews any known medication allergies, addresses anticipated difficulty in establishing an airway or aspiration risk, and prompts for placement of adequate intravenous access and availability of fluid replacement if anticipated blood loss is greater than 500 ml. Just before the skin incision, the 'Time Out'identifies the operating room team members and respective roles, and again requires verbal confirmation of the correct patient, surgical site, and procedure. Anticipated critical events are reviewed at this time including concerns from the surgeon, anesthesia team, and nurses. The 'Time Out' also reviews whether antibiotic prophylaxis has been given within the last 60 minutes and if essential imaging is displayed. Finally, at the end of the case during 'Sign Out' the nurse verbally confirms the name of the procedure to be recorded, confirms that the instrument, sponge, and needle counts are correct, and that any equipment problems that occurred during the case are appropriately addressed. Lastly, the entire surgical team including the surgeon, anesthesia team and nurses review any key concerns for the management of the patient. [2]

The concept of a 'time out' or 'surgical pause' was not necessarily new, nor was the conceptof a systematic approach to improving perioperative patient safety. In 2003 the Joint Commission Board of Commissioners approved a universal protocol which was aimed at preventing wrong site, wrong procedure, or wrong person surgery. [6] A 2006 study, in which a checklist was used in order to decrease catheter-related bloodstream infections in 108 ICUs, reported a large and sustained reduction of such infections by up to 66%. [7] However, the surgical safety checklist released by the WHO is 2008 was the first initiative of such far-reaching depth which was designed for global implementation from the earliest stages.

Implementation and Outcomes

The pilot study for the WHO's Safe Surgery Saves Lives 19 item checklist was rolled out to 8 hospitals in 8 differentcities worldwide which represented a diverse socioeconomic global population in both rural and urban areas. Data of surgical mortality and morbidity was prospectively collected between October of 2007 and September of 2008 on 3733 patients before implementation of the checklist and 3955 patients after implementation. The results published in The New England Journal of Medicine in 2009 reported a reduction in mortality from 1.5% to 0.8% and a decline in complications from 11% to 7% with both changes reaching statistical significance. Rates of surgical site infection and unplanned reoperations also significantly declined. [8] Results for urgent, noncardiac surgery were also impressive with a complication rate decrease from 18.4% to 11.7%, representing a reduction of greater than one-third. Likewise, mortality rates decreased from 3.7% to 1.4% for urgent, noncardiac surgery. [9]

After the WHO implemented the surgical checklist, marked reductions in surgical complications were reported. However, as compliance with the checklist was not complete, it was unclear whether the reported reduction in complications was due to the WHO checklist itself, or secondary to concomitant cultural shifts. In many hospitals, checklist implementation involved changes in both established healthcare delivery systems as well as in the behavior of the surgical team members. Furthermore, the implementation of such a checklist likely improved awareness of safety issues in general, as the practice of overt confirmation of correct patient identity and other safety measures were new ideas to many of the study hospitals. Thus, the idea that the observed improvements could in part be attributed simply to an increasedawareness of safety issues rather than the effect of the specific items of the checklist could be supported by the observation that during the pilot study, omission of individual items from the checklist was frequent. [8] Furthermore, the collection and documentation of patient outcomes alone likely had an effect on perioperative behavior, independent of a perioperative checklist, as in many hospitals the collection of this data was not preformed prior to these pilot studies. The nature of most of these prospective studies does not allow for participating hospitals to be blinded to the fact that they have been given a specific set of rules to follow so that data can be collected with the intent to improve patient outcomes. Thus, the Hawthorne effect likely played some role in these globally observed improvements as the participants knew they were being studied, and simply knowing this altered their behavior. Despite the inability to establish a definitive mechanism, the magnitude of reduction in surgical morbidity and mortality was impressive, and with the release of the pilot study results, countries worldwide rushed to embrace the WHO checklist for all operative procedures. [10]

During the same timeframe as the WHO pilot study, a 2008 prospective study done at the University of Toronto in Canada examined the effect of a structured surgical checklist on operating room communication. Communication errors per procedure significantly declined from 3.95 errors to 1.31 errors on average. [11] This study was one of several which were published around this same time that the WHO released their guidelines for safe surgery. At a university hospital in Finland, the authors of a study which used a modified version of WHO surgical checklist to meet national needs concluded that the implementation of the surgical checklist increased awareness of patient related issues, enhanced team communication, and prevented communication failures. [12] Thus, whether hospitals immediately adopted the new WHO guidelines in its unaltered format, adapted their own set of guidelines from the Safe Surgery Saves Lives checklist, or simply created their own de-novo checklist, it was clear that cultural changes were occurring in operating rooms across the globe.

Several follow-up studies to the WHO pilotsuggested that the impact of surgical safety checklists was highly dependent on the effectiveness of each hospital's implementation of checklist use. In one such study, when staff were not informed of how to use the checklist or why the hospital was adopting the practice, not only were staff not prepared to effectively use the list, but poor implementation also lead to frustration and eventual abandonment of the checklist despite hospital mandates. [13] In a similar study that examined predictors of successful implementation of pre- and post-operative debriefings, the authors concluded that leadership involvement at the time of the learning session was the best predictor of successful implementation of that particular safety tool. [14] Though most reports of the effectiveness of the WHO checklist implementationon reducing morbidity and mortality were positive, some follow-up studies did report impacts smaller than reported in the pilot results. One study reported a decrease in 30 day mortality from 3.13% to 2.85%, butacknowledged that the effectiveness of the checklist was highly related to compliance. [15] A prospective study that specifically examined the use of the WHO checklist on 893 orthopaedic patients failed to associate checklist use with a significant reduction in early complications or mortality despite 77% of the involved staff feeling that the checklist improved team communication. [16] Thus, despite improving perceptions of effectiveness, not all studies involving checklist use were even able to report an improvement in primary outcomes. Similarly, in a study involving 700 otorhinolaryngology patients, the authors simply concluded that the checklist improved team communication. [17]

A closer examination of the WHO pilot study of only the 4 hospitals which served areas with a higher income demographicreveals a significant reduction of death or any complication in only one of the hospitals. Surprisingly, this hospital already met 94.1% of all six WHO safety standards before checklist implementation (and 94.2% after). [10] In another one of these4 hospitals, the use of appropriate perioperative antibiotics actually declined from 98.9% to 97.6% after checklist implementation. [10] Though this effect did not reach statistical significance, it suggests that implementation of the checklist may actually worsen performance if a particular hospital already had a very effective methodology in place. In other words, in hospitals where a culture of safety was already paramount, the addition of more check boxes to a functioning system may, in fact, be counterproductive. A similar concern was addressed in a 2004 study conducted by Harvard teaching hospitals and the Massachusetts Institute of Technology in which the authors conclude that the implementation of such rigid protocols can be disabling and cause unanticipated negative consequences. Thus the authors of the latter collaborative study stress the importance of evaluating the overall impact of such protocols designed for patient safety. [18] Indeed, several studies suggest that the results of studies evaluating the use of patient safety protocols need to be interpreted with caution due to the high risk of bias in these studies [19] and the lack of consistent evidence to support their use. [20]

As previously mentioned, the concept of a checklist to improve outcomes was not a new idea for the medical sector, and its use in the medical sector has expanded beyond morbidity and mortality reductions or even a focus on safety measures. The authors of a study published in 2011 set out to determine how medical malpractice claims might be prevented by the use of a surgical checklist. The retrospective study reviewed nearly 300 surgical malpractice claims that were accepted for trial and concluded that nearly one-third of all contributing factors might have been avoided by a comprehensive surgical safety checklist. [21] Another quality improvement study published in 2012 set out to reduce negative clinical events which are related to intrahospital transfers in pediatric surgical patients by increasing communication and reinforcing feedback during these transfers. Over the course of the 1 year study involving 903 intrahospital transfers, the rate of documented problems dropped from 9.9% in the first quarter to 1% in the fourth. [22]

Conclusion

There is clear evidence that the implementation of the WHO Guidelines for Safe Surgery, whichincludes the Surgical Safety Checklist,has not only significant but dramatic positive effects in decreasing morbidity and mortality from a global perspective. However, these marked results lack a definitive mechanism. Data suggests that an increased culture of safety which developed both from the implementation of the checklist and from systematically recording outcome data may have played a larger role than the implementation of the checklist itself. However, checklist implementation specific to surgical subspecialties has been shown to correlate with significant improvements as well. Regardless, the era of safety checklist use in medicine is here, and while the systematic checking of boxes itself may not be saving lives, implementation of such practices clearly has. The practice will most definitely evolve over the coming years and likely expand to several other sectors of healthcare. The now common practice of evidenced-based medicine in the developed world has infiltrated quality improvements to become evidenced-based management. [23] Many of these methodologies are being adapted from manufacturing and other industries, such as in the case of the checklist (largely influenced by the airline industry). Though several prospective and retrospective studies are now beginning to shed light on the effects of implementation of such quality improvement methodologies, more large, multicenter, and when feasible, randomized control trials, need to be conducted in order to not only demonstrate effectiveness but to establish causality with respect to specific practices and cultural behaviors.

REFERENCES

[1] T. G. Weiser, S. E. Regenbogen, K. D. Thompson, A. B. Haynes, S. R. Lipsitz, W. R. Berry, A. A. Gawande. An estimation of the global volume of surgery: A modelling strategy based on available data. *Lancet*. 372:139-144 (2008).

[2] WHO guidelines for safe surgery. *World Alliance for Patient Safety. World Health Organization. Geneva*. (2008).

[3] WHO's patient-safety checklist for surgery. *Lancet*. 372:1 (2008).

[4] M. A. Healey, S. R. Shackford, T. M. Osler, F. B. Rogers, E. Burns. Complications in surgical patients. *Arch. Surg*. 137:611-617; discussion 617-618 (2002).

[5] *Emergency and essential surgical care*. World health organization. Geneva.Http://www.Who.Int/surgery/en/ accessed 3/5/2012.

[6] Universal protocol for preventing wrong site, wrong procedure, wrong person surgery. Joint comission. Http://www.Jointcommission.Org/ standards_information/up.Aspx accessed 3/5/12.

[7] P. Pronovost, D. Needham, S. Berenholtz, D. Sinopoli, H. Chu, S. Cosgrove, B. Sexton, R. Hyzy, R. Welsh, G. Roth, J. Bander, J. Kepros, C. Goeschel. An intervention to decrease catheter-related bloodstream infections in the icu. *N. Engl. J. Med*. 355:2725-2732 (2006).

[8] A. B. Haynes, T. G. Weiser, W. R. Berry, S. R. Lipsitz, A. H. Breizat, E. P. Dellinger, T. Herbosa, S. Joseph, P. L. Kibatala, M. C. Lapitan, A. F. Merry, K. Moorthy, R. K. Reznick, B. Taylor, A. A. Gawande. A surgical safety checklist to reduce morbidity and mortality in a global population. *N. Engl. J. Med*. 360:491-499 (2009).

[9] T. G. Weiser, A. B. Haynes, G. Dziekan, W. R. Berry, S. R. Lipsitz, A. A. Gawande. Effect of a 19-item surgical safety checklist during urgent operations in a global patient population. *Ann. Surg*. 251:976-980 (2010).

[10] C. Vijayasekar, R. J. Steele. The world health organization's surgical safety checklist. *Surgeon*. 7:260-262 (2009).

[11] L. Lingard, G. Regehr, B. Orser, R. Reznick, G. R. Baker, D. Doran, S. Espin, J. Bohnen, S. Whyte. Evaluation of a preoperative checklist and team briefing among surgeons, nurses, and anesthesiologists to reduce failures in communication. *Arch. Surg*. 143:12-17; discussion 18 (2008).

[12] R. S. Takala, S. L. Pauniaho, A. Kotkansalo, P. Helmio, K. Blomgren, M. Helminen, M. Kinnunen, A. Takala, R. Aaltonen, A. J. Katila, K. Peltomaa, T. S. Ikonen. A pilot study of the implementation of who surgical checklist in finland: Improvements in activities and communication. *Acta Anaesthesiol. Scand*. 55:1206-1214 (2011).

[13] D. M. Conley, S. J. Singer, L. Edmondson, W. R. Berry, A. A. Gawande. Effective surgical safety checklist implementation. *J. Am. Coll. Surg*. 212:873-879 (2011).

[14] D. E. Paull, L. M. Mazzia, B. S. Izu, J. Neily, P. D. Mills, J. P. Bagian. Predictors of successful implementation of preoperative briefings and postoperative debriefings after medical team training. *Am. J. Surg*. 198:675-678 (2009).

[15] W. A. van Klei, R. G. Hoff, E. E. van Aarnhem, R. K. Simmermacher, L. P. Regli, T. H. Kappen, L. van Wolfswinkel, C. J. Kalkman, W. F. Buhre, L. M. Peelen. Effects of the introduction of the who "surgical safety checklist" on in-hospital mortality: A cohort study. *Ann. Surg*. 255:44-49 (2012).

[16] M. Sewell, M. Adebibe, P. Jayakumar, C. Jowett, K. Kong, K. Vemulapalli, B. Levack. Use of the who surgical safety checklist in trauma and orthopaedic patients. *Int. Orthop*. 35:897-901 (2011).

[17] P. Helmio, K. Blomgren, A. Takala, S. L. Pauniaho, R. S. Takala, T. S. Ikonen. Towards better patient safety: Who surgical safety checklist in otorhinolaryngology. *Clin. Otolaryngol*. 36:242-247 (2011).

[18] D. MM, C. CK, R. EM, S. TB. Healthcare safety: The impact of disabling "safety" protocols. *IEEE Transactions on Systems, Man, and Cybernetics, Part A: Systems and Humans*. 34:693-698 (2004).

[19] H. C. Ko, T. J. Turner, M. A. Finnigan. Systematic review of safety checklists for use by medical care teams in acute hospital settings--limited evidence of effectiveness. *BMC Health Serv. Res*. 11:211 (2011).

[20] D. Allen, L. Rixson. How has the impact of 'care pathway technologies' on service integration in stroke care been measured and what is the strength of the evidence to support their effectiveness in this respect? *Int. J. Evid. Based Healthc*. 6:78-110 (2008).

[21] E. N. de Vries, M. P. Eikens-Jansen, A. M. Hamersma, S. M. Smorenburg, D. J. Gouma, M. A. Boermeester. Prevention of surgical malpractice claims by use of a surgical safety checklist. *Ann. Surg*. 253:624-628 (2011).

[22] D. K. Nakayama, S. S. Lester, D. R. Rich, B. C. Weidner, J. B. Glenn, I. J. Shaker. Quality improvement and patient care checklists in intrahospital transfers involving pediatric surgery patients. *J. Pediatr. Surg*. 47:112-118 (2012).

[23] C. R. Nicolay, S. Purkayastha, A. Greenhalgh, J. Benn, S. Chaturvedi, N. Phillips, A. Darzi. Systematic review of the application of quality improvement methodologies from the manufacturing industry to surgical healthcare. *Br. J. Surg*. 99:324-335 (2012).

In: Quality Improvement
Editors: K. W. Lobdell and S. C. Stamou
ISBN: 978-1-62417-390-5

Chapter 8

Quality Assurance and Technical Performance in the Operating Room

***John M. Karamichalis*[1] *and Pedro del Nido*[2]**
[1]Division of Pediatric Cardiothoracic Surgery, Department of Surgery, University of California San Francisco, San Francisco, CA, US
[2]Department of Cardiac Surgery, Children's Hospital Boston and Harvard Medical School, Boston, MA, US

Abstract

Outcomes in pediatric cardiac surgery have improved dramatically since its infancy 50 years ago. Mortality has been reduced from as high as 90-100% in the initial years to around 4% for many high complexity cases and virtually no mortality for simple cardiac defects. While part of this improvement can be attributed to advances in pediatric cardiac anesthesia, pediatric cardiopulmonary bypass and development of highly specialized pediatric cardiac intensive care units, outcomes continue to depend on the technical quality of the surgical repair. In this article we address the importance of the surgical technical performance on outcomes and discuss the currently available tools for measurement of surgical competency. Our studies showed that the final technical (anatomical) result score had the strongest association with patient outcomes. We offer suggestions for a competency model that continues to evolve as we explore the use of immersive learning, deliberate practice, reflection in action, mentorship by senior surgeons and life long learning. We expand our discussion to include the applicability of such a quality assurance tool in adult cardiac surgery.

Keywords: Surgical competency, pediatric cardiac surgery, technical performance, risk stratification, outcomes, patient safety

Introduction

Advances over the last two decades in the understanding, diagnosis and surgical treatment of congenital cardiac lesions have resulted in mortality reduced from 100% forty years ago to around 4% for many highly complex cases to almost 0% for low complexity cases [1]. The increased awareness of the advances in this field have led to greater expectations from the public and medical community. In addition, the current evolution of health care towards performance based reimbursements (i.e. Pay-for-Performance) along with the implementation of several quality control and improvement programs have resulted in increased scrutiny and monitoring of surgical competencies and outcomes in pediatric cardiac surgery.

Surgical competence in pediatric cardiac surgery is very difficult to quantify or measure directly since patient survival or physiologic status post repair, the most commonly reported endpoints, often are determined by multiple factors.A quantifiable metric is highly desirable for purposes of surgeon self assessment and to determine the impact of surgical performance on patient outcome and overall institutional performance. One very important feature of such a metricis the ability to distinguish between an individual surgeon's competence and an entire congenital heart program's performance. An individual practitioner's surgical performance includes the technical domain and other non-technical skills such as cognitive flexibility, decision making, anticipation, situational awareness, communication team work and leadership [29-31]. This chapter will focus on the individual surgeons' technical performance.

Until recently, hospital mortality, often in the form of cumulative sum (cusum) analysis, had been used as a surrogate measure of technical performance in congenital heart surgery [2-4]. Raw mortality data, however, do not correct for the case complexity or other associated factors that might affect outcomes. One alternative, the Hospital Standardized Mortality Ratio (HSMR) is intended as an overall measure of deaths in hospital, a proportion of which will be preventable. High ratios may thus suggest potential problems with quality of care [5]. The HSMR is a complex, but inexpensive and a relatively easy method to calculate from national or other benchmark data the patients' predicted risks of death. However, there are a number of methodological challenges in HMSR's construction and interpretation, in large part due to the fact that they are based on administrative databases [6].

While risk-adjusted in-hospital death rates may be a reasonable measure of institutional performance, this measure is inadequate to assess the performance of individual practitioners due to the many additional factors such as the contribution and impact of other team members, outside the control of an individual surgeon. This is especially problematic for high risk operations, which require a complex multi-departmental microsystem consisting of dedicated teams composed of many individuals and specialties.

Finding ways to evaluate, monitor and improve surgical competency becomes important in improving outcomes in pediatric cardiac surgery (PCS). It is imperative first to define optimal or acceptable surgical performance. There is little available data on the importance of technical performance in determining outcomes independent of the anatomic factors and perioperative care management. Although risk-adjusted mortality evaluations allow for a better understanding than general mortality rates, they are not intended to evaluate individual competency or performance. Furthermore, congenital heart surgeons have few available tools for systematic self-assessment as part of an on-going quality improvement evaluation process. While outcomes are dependent on multiple factors including the patient's underlying pathology, case complexity, age, physiologic status, healthcare delivery systems, technical performance defined as *the adequacy of the surgical anatomic repair intended*is an important component in this evaluation. [11-16].

We previouslydevelopeda method to measure surgical technical performance for congenital heart disease as part of a quality improvement evaluation process to be used for peer self-assessment [7-10]. This was initially piloted in selected surgical procedures including repairs of ventricular septal defect, tetralogy of Fallot, complete common atrioventricularseptal defects, arterial switch operation and the stage I Norwood procedure [7-9], which was then expanded to include most operations in infants [10] and most recently expanded to include almost all operations in congenital cardiac surgery [26]. This work demonstrated that technical performance defined as the adequacy of the anatomic repair, can be assessed in congenital heart surgery and the implementation of a technical performance scoring system covering the majority of congenital cardiac surgery operations is feasible. Technical performance scores correlate with early outcomes all across the spectrum of congenital cardiac surgery and especially in the high complexity operations such as the stage I Norwood procedure. Technical excellence during surgery, with little to insignificant residual defects, has the best outcomes along the entire spectrum of case complexity. This was particularly important in determining outcomes as case complexity increased [9-10]. The impact of less than optimal technical scores depended on the risk category,with higher mortality in the higher risk patients and longer ventilation times and ICU and hospital length of stay, with likely increased resource utilization for the lower risk group [26].

Surgical Competency and Technical Performance

The assessment of surgical competency, remains an elusive concept. Surgeons must possess specific competencies defined as the knowledge, skills and attitudes (KSA) such as the ability to exchange information and coordinate individual team members [12]. Surgical technical competency is the ability of the surgical microsystem to successfully and safely execute the necessary steps in order to perform a specific operation for a patient [11]. KSA deficiencies can be recognized using reliable and valid measures, and support, accurate feedback can be provided, and appropriate instructional strategies for remediation can be selected and implemented. When done on a regular basis, this deliberate practice, can lead to sustained expertise and standards [25]. While the precise execution of the technical aspects of an operation is an important component of surgical competency, surgical competency encompasses many more team skills and attitudes beyond the technical maneuvers required in surgery. These include: (a) team interaction and leadership both pre-, intra- and post-operatively: (b) decision making ensuring that the right operation is selected and performed; and, (c) delivery of timely information to the patients family and other health care providers [13].

Surgical excellence, beyond excellent three-dimensional perception, ability to restructure cardiac and vascular anatomy to enable visualization of key anatomic features, and manual dexterity involves less measurable aspects such as the ability to prevent or deal with complications, understand cardiovascular physiology, cardiopulmonary bypass and myocardial protection, aswell as address and mitigate the impact of human factors components such as fatigue, situational awareness, decision making skills, multitasking and prioritizing [14-16].

Development of Technical Performance Scoring Tool

The concept of assessing the technical performance of surgeons in congenital cardiac surgery, defined as the adequacy of anatomic repair, was recently introduced at Boston

Children's Hospital in Massachusetts. The technical steps leading to the anatomic repair of a lesion are mostly under the control of the surgeon. Intraoperative technical performance is one of the most important aspects of the therapeutic process and determines patient outcomes especially in high acuity operations [9,10,17,18].

This tool was designed to be used for peer and self-assessment as none of the currently available quality monitoring tools measures technical performance per se. It was initially piloted in selected surgical procedures including repairs of ventricular septal defect, tetralogy of Fallot, complete common atrioventricular canal, arterial switch and later the stage I Norwood procedure [7-9].

The use was then expanded to include a variety of other operations [10] and more recently to cover almost the entire spectrum of congenital cardiac surgery operations [26]. The score was created by dividing the surgical procedure into individual components defined as sub-procedures, which are based on the specific anatomic regions subject to the surgical intervention (please see Table 1 examples for a VSD repair, an arterial switch operation and a stage I Norwood operation).

The parameters of the score assessment were defined and piloted by a modified delphi consensus process of cardiologists and cardiac surgeons. The score was based primarily on pre-discharge echocardiographic measurements but also on cardiac catheterization data, the need for post-operative catheterization laboratory or operating room based re-interventions. The technical tool defined three possible categories for each sub-procedure: *"optimal", "adequate" and "inadequate"*. An overall summary score for the main surgical procedure was also defined, wherein the operation was graded as *optimal* if all the sub-procedures were optimal; *adequate*, if the sub-procedures were optimal or adequate, but none inadequate; and *inadequate,* if one or more sub-procedures were inadequate.

The anatomic regions operated on were scored by subdividing the complex procedures into basic components where each component of a given repair was scrutinized and analyzed separately. The technical performance of a given surgeon that closed a VSD, for example, was not just studied by looking at the technical score for isolated VSD procedures but rather all VSDs repaired by the surgeon, including those associated with other repaired defects, would be included in the technical analysis, thus increasing the statistical reliability of the assessment.

The initial pilot study demonstrated that despite PCS procedural diversity and complexity, the adequacy of the surgical repair can be assessed using a reliable technical performance scoring system. The main limitation of the assessment of technical performance is that it is primarily based on echocardiography, an operator-dependent technique with well known limitations [19]. These limitations include the assessment of aortic arch gradients, valve gradients and repair, aortopulmonary shunt patency, and the dependency on thoracic windows. Conversely, for a scoring system to be widely used simplicity and reliability are key factors. Echocardiography fulfills this criterion because it is a bedside test that is widely available and has proven valid and reliable as a stand-alone test in the preoperative and postoperative evaluation of children with congenital heart lesions. Furthermore, in most congenital centers, it is routinely used intra-operatively and/or prior to discharge. However, in order to make echocardiography a useful tool for objective assessment of adequacy of surgical repair, standardization of views and measurement parameters is required. This aspect of the Technical Performance Score also requires consensus amongst echocardiographers. Fortunately, most trans-thoracic echo views are now standard across most centers, and there are generally agreed upon findings for quantitative and semi-quantitative evaluation of residual lesions.

Table 1. Examples of Technical performance scoring criteria

a. Ventricular Septal Defect repair*

Subprocedures	Optimal	Adequate	Inadequate
ASD repair	No or trivial residual shunt (1mm)	Small residual shunt 2-3 mm	Reintervention*or* Residual shunt >3 mm
VSD repair, membranous	No or trivial residual shunt (1mm)	Residual defect 2-3 mm	Reintervention*or* Residual defect >3 mm
VSD closure, muscular	No or trivial residual shunt (1mm)	Residual defect 2-3 mm	Reintervention*or* Residual defect >3 mm
PDA closure	No residual PDA	Residual PDA 1 mm	Reintervention*or* Residual defect >1 mm
Conduction	Normal conduction No change from pre-op	Normal conduction No change from pre-op	Need for permanent Pacemaker

*Modified from reference [7].

b. Arterial Switch Operation

Subprocedures	Optimal	Adequate	Inadequate
ASD repair, secundum	No or trivial residual shunt 1mm	Small residual defect (2-3 mm)	Reintervention*or* Residual shunt >3 mm
VSD repair	No or trivial residual shunt 1mm	Small residual defect (2-3 mm)	Reintervention*or* Residual shunt >3 mm
VSD repair, muscular	No or trivial residual shunt 1mm	Small residual defect (2-3 mm)	Reintervention*or* Residual shunt >3 mm
Pulmonary outflow tract repair	No residual gradient (peak Gradient <15 mmHg)	Mild gradient 15-30 mm Hg	Reintervention*or* Gradient >30 mm Hg
PA reconstruction (plasty), branch	No or trivial branch PA narrowing or gradient (peak gradient <15 mmHg)	Mild narrowing Mild residual gradient 15-30 mm Hg	Reintervention*or* Gradient >30 mm Hg Branch PA *z* score <-3
Systemic outflow tract repair	No or trivial gradient (peak <15 mmHg)	Mild gradient 15-30 mm Hg	Reintervention*or* Gradient >30 mm Hg
Coronaries reimplantation	No obstruction to coronary flow	No obstruction to coronary flow	Reintervention Coronary flow compromise, ischemia/infarction, with echo and/or ECG findings
Aortic Arch (when applicable)	No or trivial gradient peak<15 mmHg	Mild gradient 15-30 mmHg	Reintervention Moderate to severe gradient. Gradient >30mmHg based on echo
Relief of RVOT obstruction (when applicable)	No or trivial residual obstruction, peak gradient <15 mmHg	Mild residual gradient 15-30 mm Hg	Reintervention*or* Gradient >30 mm Hg
Conduction	Normal conduction No change from pre-op	Normal conduction No change from pre-op	Need for permanent pacemaker

*Modified from reference [7].

c. Stage I. Norwood operation

Subprocedures	Optimal	Adequate	Inadequate
Proximal arch reconstruction	No or trivial gradient <10 mmHg No evidence of coronary ischemia	Mild peak gradient at proximal aortopulmonary anastomosis or proximal arch gradient 10-25mmHg (echo or cath)	Need for reintervention during initial hospital stay More than mild gradient >25 mm Hg (echo or cath)
Distal arch reconstruction	No or trivial narrowing or flow acceleration by echo peak gradient<15 mmHg	Mild gradient 15-30 mmHg (by echo orcath)	Need for reintervention during initial hospital stay Peak gradient > 30 mmHg (echo or cath)
Coronary perfusion	Unobstructed flow into proximal coronary arteries	Unobstructed flow into proximal coronary arteries	Need for reintervention during initial hospital stay Evidence for obstructed coronary flow (eg echo, cath, EKG)
Atrial septectomy	No or trivial gradient mean gradient 1-2 mmHg Restrictive atrial septum left on purpose	Mean gradient 3-4 mm Hg (unless intended)	Need for reintervention during initial hospital stay Mean gradient > 4 mm Hg (unless intended)
Source of pulmonary blood flow			
a. Modified BT shunt	Patent	Patent Downsizing of shunt because of pulmonary overcirculation	Need of reintervention for or presence of kinking, clot, obstruction/distortion of the BT shunt or the Branch PAs)
b. RV-PA conduit	Patent	Patent Downsizing of shunt because of pulmonary overcirculation	Need of reintervention for or presence of: kinking, clot, obstruction/distortion of the BT shunt or the Branch PAs)

* Modified from reference [8].

Technical Performance and Outcomes

Subsequent studies have demonstrated a strong impact of technical performance on hospital survival in patients undergoing stage I Norwood procedure [8,9]. Avoiding a technically inadequate outcome was a major determinant of patient survival. This indicates that technical scores could be an especially useful tool to improve surgical performance by offering reflective feedback that would help to reduce morbidity in high complexity operations. Furthermore, low mortality rates were observed in the optimal category suggesting that excellent technical results are necessary for survival; however, they may not be sufficient for good patient outcomes, especially in the highly complex cohort.A large role is also likely played by other factors such as structural or procedural factors or patient specific risk factors such as patient's weight, prematurity, chromosomal anomalies, the presence of preoperative shock or poor physiological status, etc.

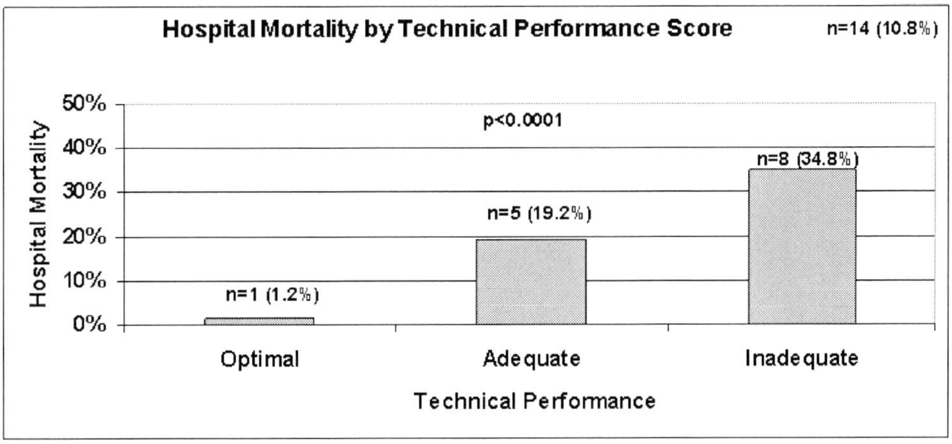

*Modified from reference [9].

Figure 1a*.

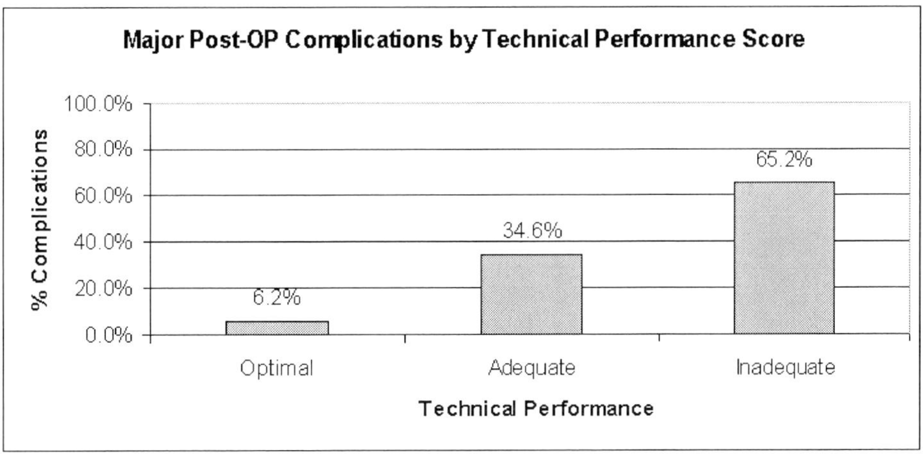

*Modified from reference [9].

Figure 1b*.

While the previous studies demonstrated that technical performance has a major effect on outcomes after stage I Norwood operations, the interplay of baseline physiologic status, anatomic risk factors, and technical performance was subsequently studied [9]. The association of preoperative baseline physiology was measured using the Pediatric Risk of Mortality III scoring system (PRISM III), case complexity was measured by Aristotle comprehensive score, and the technical performance and outcomes were defined following the stage I Norwood procedure. The study confirmed previous findings and demonstrated a significant association between preoperative physiologic illness severity score (as measured by PRISM III and partially by Aristotle), case complexity measured by the Aristotle score, technical performance and patient outcomes. Optimal technical performance attenuated the impact of preoperative illness severity and resulted in better outcomes regardless of the pre-operative illness severity or case complexity.

Notably, inadequate technical performance resulted in poor outcomes regardless of the preoperative illness severity or case complexity. Specifically, patients with optimal technical scores undergoing the stage I Norwood procedure had an overall 1.2% in-hospital mortality versus 34.8% in those with inadequate technical scores [9] (Figure 1a). Patients with inadequate performance scores had significantly longer hospital and ICU stays, longer ventilation times and a greater occurrence of major post-operative complications ($p<0.0001$ for each comparison) [9], Figure 1b.

An adequate technical performance resulted in better outcomes for lower preoperative illness severity or case complexity and poorer outcomes for higher preoperative illness severity or case complexity (see Figure 2). In other words, the clinical outcomes for patients with adequate technical performance were dictated by their baseline physiology and anatomy, whereas, the outcomes for patients with optimal or inadequate performance were dependent more on the actual technical results, rather than on the baseline physiology or anatomy. The technical performance had the highest predictive value for patient outcomes. Specifically, the receiver operating characteristic (ROC) analysis showed significant ability of technical performance scores to discriminate mortality, with an area under the curve of 0.84 ($p<0.001$;95% CI, 0.74-0.94) illustrating the impact of sound intraoperative technique. The technical performance emerged as a powerful predictor of clinical outcomes for stage I Norwood operation.

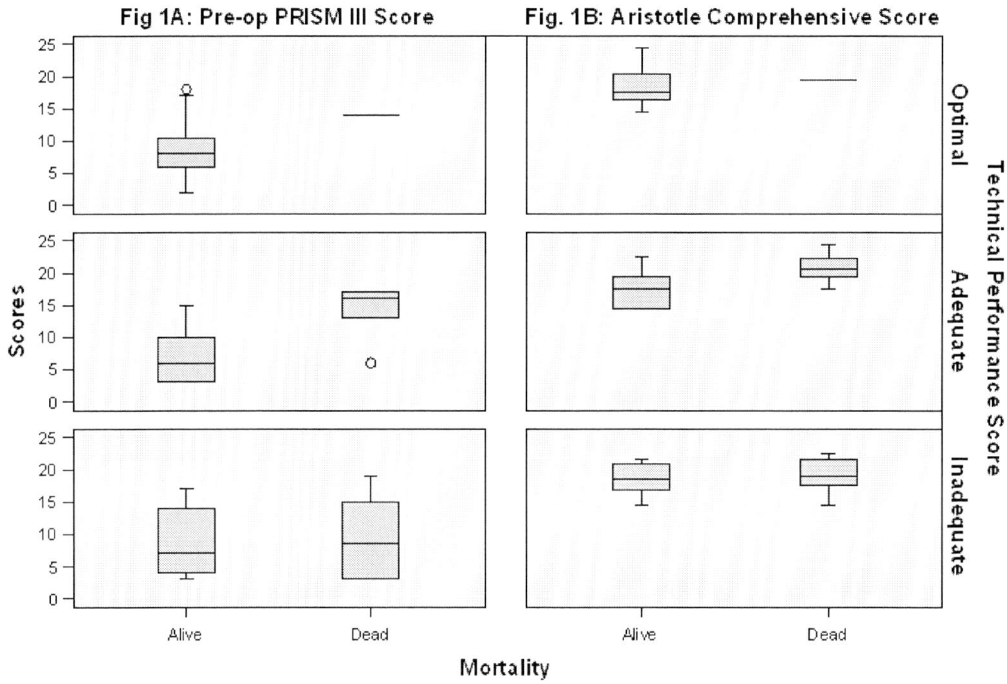

*Modified from reference [9].

Figure 2.* Subgroup analysis measured by technical performance score and peri-operative physiologic status (measured by PRISM III score) or case complexity (measured by Aristotle score) versus mortality in stage I Norwood procedure.

Risk Stratification

Risk adjustment is critical in considering the underlying risks of taking care of sick patients. Risk adjustment is essential to avoid penalizing clinicians and institutions treating complex cases. The main risk adjustment systems such as the Risk Assessment in Congenital Heart Surgery -1 (RACHS-1), the Aristotle Basic and Comprehensive complexity scoring system, and the newly developed European Association of Cardiothoracic Surgery–Society of Thoracic Surgeons (EACTS-STS) system are aimed at risk stratifying outcomes based on the case complexity of the operation [20,21], and in the latter on the actual reported mortality in a large cohort of patients across many institutions. These scoring systems take into consideration other factors such as the anatomic and physiological status, age, prematurity, and genetic anomalies. This enables a standardized analysis of outcomes between different surgeons and centers after adjusting for case mix and risk.

Risk adjustment is a challenge that is not addressed by the presently used technical scores. Should a technical score include patient-specific non-modifiable risk factors? These might include factors such as the weight or prematurity, as is typically done in clinical performance risk-adjusted methods such as RACHS-1, or Aristotle system, or should it include only technique-specific anatomic risk factors such as a single papillary muscle in complete atrioventricularseptal defect or anomalous coronary arteries in an Arterial Switch Operation? Some kind of risk adjustment is therefore necessary in the interpretation of technical scores in operations that are of different case complexity or acuity.

Technical Performance and Post-operative Physiologic Illness Severity

Technical performance was demonstrated to have a significant impact on postoperative physiologic illness severity when measured by PRISM III, with higher PRISM III scores associated with inadequate performance [8]. The severity of illness as measured by the PRISM III on the first post-operative day after a stage I Norwood operation, had a high association and discrimination in regards to hospital mortality, postoperative re-intervention, inadequate technical performance and the occurrence of major postoperative complications. The PRISM III therefore may be used as an early surrogate of technical performance and it could be used to initiate a timely search for technical deficiencies the institution of supportive measures and re-interventions to address them.

Technical Performance Predicts Post-operative Morbidity

The technical performance score was one of the main predictors of postoperative morbidity in a prospective study of 166 neonates and infants (less than 6 months of age) undergoing a wide variety of low and high complexity heart surgery [10]. Optimal technical scores predicted low post-operative adverse events. Adequate technical scores were associated with higher post-operative morbidity in patients with higher case complexity and lower morbidity in those with lower case complexity (see Figure 3). Notably, inadequate technical scores were associated with higher morbidity irrespective of case complexity. The patient outcomes were not affected by intra-operative adverse events, such as re-institution of cardiopulmonary bypass and surgical revisions, provided technical performance score was at least adequate [10].

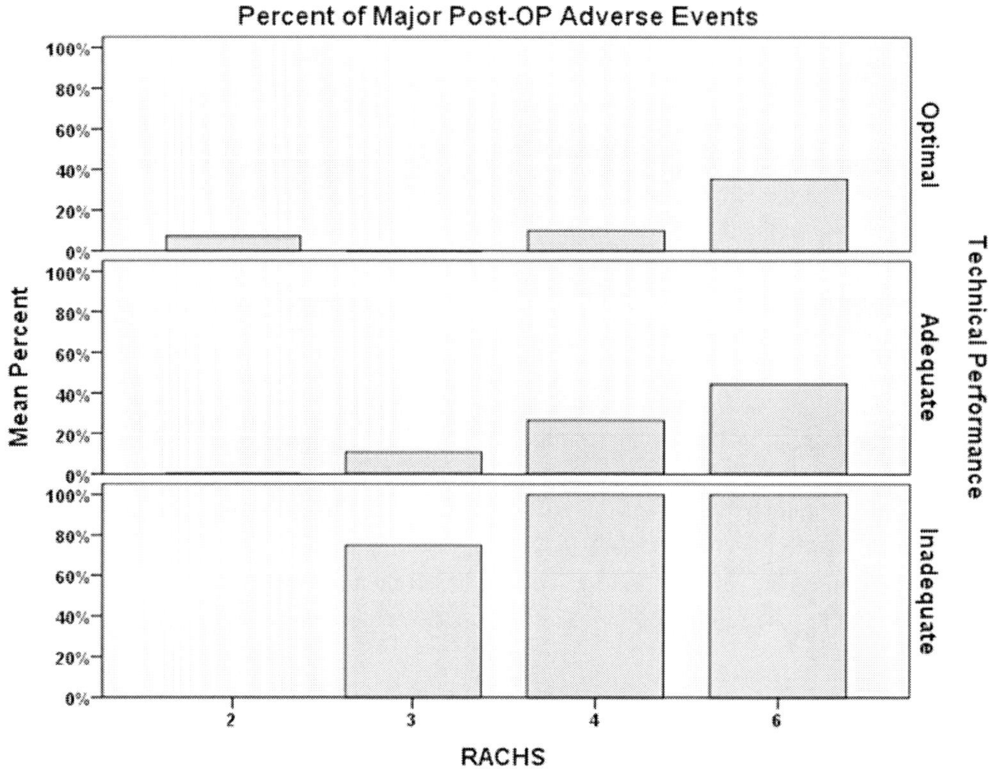

* Modified from reference 10.
RACHS, Risk Adjustment in Congenital Heart Surgery. Post-OP=postoperative.

Figure 3.* Major postoperative adverse events based on technical scores and RACHS-1 categories for 166 patients less than 6 months of age undergoing heart surgery. This Figure outlines the percentage of patients with major postoperative adverse events comparing the technical performance and RACHS-1 risk categories. Optimal technical performance had a low occurrence of adverse events, whereas adequate technical performance had low rates of events in the low complexity groups (RACHS-1 categories 2 and 3, but higher percentage of adverse events in the higher risk categories (RACHS-1 categories 4 and 6). Inadequate technical performance had the highest percentage with adverse events in all categories of the RACHS-1 system.

An important point is that none of our studies showed that longer cross clamp times were associated with worse outcomes [8-10]. In the past, the focus on "speedy surgery" and short cross-clamp times had dominated the thinking and has lead to shortcuts and a reluctance to go back and fix problems for fear of ventricular dysfunction due to long ischemic times. The final technical (anatomical) result scores had the strongest association with patient outcomes [15,16,22,23]. With excellent cardioplegia solutions available nowadays and refined myocardial protection and cardiopulmonary bypass methods, the myocardial ischemic time (i.e. cross clamp time) is a lesser factor that impacts clinical outcomes to a significant degree.

Technical Performance Scores in the Operating Room

Our studies underscore the importance of what is called "technical imperative", an absolute rule whereby it is imperative for patients to leave the operating room with a good or better yet optimal result. While our proposed system above is based primarily on technical scores based on the pre-discharge echo results and the need of post-operative re-interventions, it is obvious that the assessment of technical performance is of paramount importance to be done in the operating room, prior to the patient leaving the operating table and any residual lesions corrected. We demonstrated [10] that the outcomes of complex congenital cardiac operations are not affected by intraoperative adverse events, including surgical revisions, provided technical performance score is at least adequate underscoring the importance of "technical imperative". In addition a more recent study [28] demonstrated that technical performance affects midterm survival following infant cardiac surgery. Inadequate technical performance scores can be used to prospectively identify patients at risk for ongoing demise and need for re-interventions, concluding that an aggressive approach to diagnosing and treating residual lesions at initial operation is warranted.

The assessment of the technical adequacy of the anatomic repair can be performed in the operating room using a variety of proposed methods with the deliberate use of intraoperative transesophageal and epicardial echo assessment of the repair, with the adjunct use of hemodynamic measurements and direct visual observations in the completing a full picture of the adequacy of the repair. The prompt assessment of technical performance in the operating room has the advantage of providing important information to the operating surgeon, which can aid in deciding whether to go back on bypass and repair any residual lesions.

Conclusion

The comprehensive assessment of surgical competency remains an elusive though important concept. The continued performance monitoring of congenital cardiac surgeons is vital and might one day become a requirement of national boards and regulators as a quality control measurement. Our studies have shown that technical performance has emerged as an important predictor of outcomes in congenital surgery. We describe a "technical imperative", defined as an absolute rule whereby it is imperative to leave the operating room with a good or better yet, an optimal technical result, even if this requires surgical revision and going back on bypass [8,9,10,17]. Cross clamp times were not associated with poor outcomes but rather it was the end result of the adequacy of anatomic repair that counted the most. Thus, a focus on the intraoperative assessment of the adequacy of the anatomic repairprimarily by echocardiography but also by pressure measurements and even intraoperative angiography is paramount. Increasing intraoperative vigilance, the detection and immediate repair of significant residual lesions remains of prime importance.

Our studies also indicate that residual defects repaired in a timely fashion, which usually means immediately in the operating room, or within 24 hours of surgery result in no significant impact on patient outcome, even in high complexity cases.

The development and implementation of a system for measuring technical performance in congenital cardiac surgery operations can be used for surgeons' self and peer assessment. The use of the technical score in conjunction with a risk adjustment system such as RACHS-1, Aristotle or EACTS-STS, was found to be a useful tool in quality improvement and the monitoring of surgical performance. The assessment of surgical performance in the operating room could be expanded and applied to adult cardiac surgery operations using the same principles. Eventhough our methodology was exclusively applied to congenital cardiac surgery operations, this system is applicable in adult cardiac surgery, and may be applicable to non-cardiac procedures as well. The intraoperative and deliberate use of different tools and methods such as transesophageal echocardiography, hemodynamic measurements, visual inspection in assessing the adequacy of the anatomic repair while the patient is still on the operating table is of paramount importance in cardiac surgery.

We have proposed a model of assessing technical performance in congenital heart surgery that is focused primarily on the outcome and the adequacy of the anatomic repair that is felt to be under the surgeon's control.

This system permits individual surgeons to self-assess technical performance and provide specific benchmarks which can lead to the development of technical performance metrics in the operating room to develop national benchmarks. The system does not preclude the use of other quality metrics in evaluating the surgeon's performance, which should include leadership skills, and ability to communicate and function effectively within a multidisciplinary team. These other factors may turn out to be just as important in determining patient outcomes and providing quality assurance measures which are of paramount importance in ensuring excellent patient care in cardiac surgery.

References

[1] Congenital Heart Disease: A Surgical-Historical Perspective, Castaneda, *Ann of Thorac Surgery* 2006: 79, S2217-20.

[2] Stark J. F., Gallivan S., Davis K., Hamilton J. R. L., Monro J. L., Pollock J. C. S., Watterson K. G. Assessment of mortality rates for congenital heart defects and surgeons' performance. *Ann. Thorac. Surg.,* Jul 2001; 72: 169 - 175.

[3] Welke K. F., Karamlou T., Ungerleider R. M., Diggs B. S. Mortality rate is not a valid indicator of quality differences between pediatric cardiac surgical programs. *Ann Thorac Surg.* 2010 Jan;89(1):139-44; discussion 145-6.

[4] Welke K. F., Diggs B. S., Karamlou T., Ungerleider R. M. The relationship between hospital surgical case volumes and mortality rates in pediatric cardiac surgery: a national sample, 1988-2005. *Ann Thorac Surg.* 2008 Sep;86(3):889-96; discussion 889-96.

[5] Jarman B., Gault S., Alves B., Hider A., Dolan S., Cook A. et al. Explaining differences in English hospital death rates using routinely collected data. *BMJ* 1999;318:1515-20.

[6] Mohammed M. A., Deeks J. J., Girling A., Rudge G., Carmalt M., Stevens A. J., Lilford R. J. Evidence of methodological bias in hospital standardised mortality ratios: Retrospective database study of English hospitals. *BMJ.* 2009 Mar 18;338:b780. doi: 10.1136/bmj.b780. Erratum in: BMJ. 2009 Apr 1. doi: 10.1136/bmj.b1348.

[7] Larrazabal L. A., del Nido P. J., Jenkins K. J., Gauvreau K., Lacro S., Colan S. D., Pigula F., Benavidez O. J., Fynn-Thompson F., Mayer J. E., Bacha E. A: Measurement of technical performance in congenital heart surgery:A pilot study: *Ann Thorac Surg* 2007;83:179-84.

[8] Bacha E. A., Larrazabal L. A., Pigula F. A., Gauvreau K., Jenkins K. J., Colan S. D., Fynn-Thompson F., Mayer J. E., del Nido P. J. Measurement of technical performance

in surgery for congenital heart disease: The stage I Norwood procedure. *J Thora cCardiovasc Surg*. 2008; 136:993-7.

[9] Karamichalis J. M., Thiagarajan R. R., Liu H., Mamic P., Gauvreau K., Bacha E. A. Stage I Norwood: Optimal Technical Performance improves outcomes irrespective of pre-operative physiologic status or case-complexity. *J Thorac Cardiovasc Surg* 2010;139:962-968.

[10] Nathan M., Karamichalis J., Liu H., del Nido P., Pigula F.,Thiagarajan R., Bacha E. A. Intra-operative adverse events can be compensated in infants after cardiac surgery: A prospective study. *J Thorac. Cardiovasc. Surg.* Aug 2011 in press.

[11] Mohr, J., Batalden, P., Barach, P. Integrating Patient Safety into the Clinical Microsystem, *Quality and Safety in Healthcare* 2004;13:34-38.

[12] Barach, P., Weinger, M. *Trauma Team Performance*. In: Trauma: Emergency Resuscitation and Perioperative Anesthesia Management., Vol 1,Wilson, W. C., Grande, C.M. Hoyt, D.B. (Eds.), Marcel Dekker, Inc. 2007, 101-113. NY. ISBN: 10-0-8247-2916-6.

[13] Baker, D. Battles J, King H, Salas, E., Barach, P. The Role of Teamwork in the Professional Education of Physicians: Current Status and Assessment Recommendations. *Joint Commission Journal on Qualityand Safety2005*; 31:4:185-202.

[14] Schraagen J. M., Schouten A., Smit M., van der Beek D., Van de Ven J. Barach P. A prospective study of paediatric cardiac surgical microsystems: Assessing the relationships between non-routine events, teamwork and patient outcomes; *BMJ Qual Saf 2011*. doi:10.1136/ bmjqs.2010.048983.

[15] Catchpole K. R., Giddings A. E., de Leval M. R. et al. Identification of systems failures in successful paediatric cardiac surgery. *Ergonomics* 2006;49:567e88.

[16] Arthey J., deLeval M., Reason J. T. The human factor in cardiac surgery: errors and near misses in a high technology medical domain. *Ann Thorac Surg* 2001;72:300e5.

[17] Karamichalis J. M., del Nido P. J., Thiagarajan R. R., Liu H., Gauvreau K., Pigula F. A., Fynn-Thompson F. E., Emani S. M., Mayer J. E. Jr., Bacha E. A. Early post-operative severity of illness predicts outcomes following the stage I Norwood procedure. *Ann Thorac Surg* 2011; 92:660-665.

[18] NathanM., Karamichalis J. M., Liu H., Mayer J. E. Jr., Fynn-Thompson F., Emani S., del Nido P.,Pigula F., Thiagarajan R., Bacha E. A. Technical Performance of the Repair, But Not Intraoperative Adverse Events, Is a Powerful Predictor Oral presentation at the *Congenital Heart Surgeons Society Annual Meeting, Chicago, IL* October 24-25, 2010.

[19] Vlahos A. P., Marx G. R., McElhinney D., Oneill S., Goudevenos I., Colan S. D. Clinical utility of Doppler Echocardiography in assessing aortic stenosis severity and predicting need for intervention in children. *PediatrCardiol.* 2008 May;29(3):507-14.

[20] O'Brien S. M., Clarke D. R., Jacobs J. P., Jacobs M. L., Lacour-Gayet F. G., Pizarro C., Welke K. F., Maruszewski B., Tobota Z., Miller W. J., Hamilton L., Peterson E. D., Mavroudis C., Edwards F. H. An empirically based tool for analyzing mortality associated with congenital heart surgery. *J ThoracCardiovasc Surg.* 2009 Nov;138(5):1139-53.

[21] Jacobs M. L., Jacobs J. P., Jenkins K. J., Gauvreau K., Clarke D. R., Lacour-Gayet F. Stratification of complexity: the Risk Adjustment for Congenital Heart Surgery-1 method and the Aristotle Complexity Score--past, present, and future. *Cardiol Young.* 2008 Dec;18 Suppl 2:163-8.

[22] Barach P., Johnson J. K., Ahmad A., Galvan C., Bognar A., Duncan R., Starr J. P., Bacha E. A. A prospective observational study of human factors, adverse events, and patient outcomes in surgery for pediatric cardiac disease. *J ThoracCardiovasc Surg.* 2008 Dec;136(6):1422-8. Epub 2008 Sep 6.

[23] de Leval M. R., Carthey J., Wright D. J., Farewell V. T., Reason J. T. Human factors and cardiac surgery: a multicenter study. *J ThoracCardiovasc Surg.* 2000 Apr;119(4 Pt 1):661-72.

[24] Australian Institue of Health and Welfare. *Australia's Children. TheirHealth and Welfare*. Canberra: AIHW2002.

[25] Ericsson, Anders K.; Charness, Neil; Feltovich, Paul; Hoffman, Robert R. (2006). *Cambridge handbook on expertise and expert performance*. Cambridge, UK: Cambridge University Press.

[26] Karamichalis J. M., Colan S. D., Nathan M., Pigula F. A., Baird C., Marx G., Emani S. M., Geva T., Fynn-Thompson F. E., Liu H., Mayer J. E. Jr., del Nido, P. J. Technical Performance Scores in Congenital Cardiac Surgery: A Quality Assessment Initiative. *Ann Thorac Surg* 2012;94:1317-23.

[27] Karamichalis J. M., BarachP.,Nathan M., Henaine R., del Nido P. J., Bacha E: Assessment of Technical Competency in Pediatric Cardiac Surgery. *Progress in Pediatric Cardiology* 2012;33:15-20.

[28] Nathan M., Karamichalis J. M., Liu H., Emani S., Baird C., Pigula F., Colan S., Thiagarajan R., Bacha E., del Nido P. Surgical Technical Performance Scores are predictors for late mortality and unplanned reinterventions in infants after cardiac surgery. *J Thorac Cardiovasc Surg* 2012;144:1095-1101.

[29] Yule S., Flin R., Paterson-Brown S., Maran N., Rowley D. Development of a rating system for surgeons' non-technical skills. *Med Educ* 2006 Nov:40(11):1098-104.

[30] Giddings A. E. B., Williamson C. *The Leadership and Management ofSurgical Teams*. The Royal College of Surgeons of England, June 2007. (www.Rcseng.ac.uk/publications/docs/leadership_management. html).

[31] Baker, D. Battles J., King H., Salas, E., Barach, P. The Role of Teamwork in the Professional Education of Physicians: Current Status and Assessment Recommendations. *Joint Commission Journal on Qualityand Safety 2005*; 31:4:185-202.

In: Quality Improvement
Editors: K. W. Lobdell and S. C. Stamou
ISBN: 978-1-62417-390-5

Chapter 9

Collaboration in Cardiac Surgical Quality Improvement: The Virginia Experience

Edwin Fonner, Jr., Alan M. Speir and Jeffrey B. Rich
Virginia Cardiac Surgery Quality Initiative, VA, US

Abstract

The Virginia Cardiac Surgery Quality Initiative (VCSQI) is a voluntary, self-funded non-profit collaboration of 17 hospitals and 13 cardiac surgical practices in the Commonwealth of Virginia. The group facilitates collaboration between hospitals and physicians in order to improve clinical quality across an entire state in programs of all sizes through data sharing, outcomes analysis, and process improvements. This is a multi-site, multidisciplinary membership alliance that performs 99% of the open-heart surgical procedures in the state. All members of the surgical team participate in meetings and quality initiatives. The group's extended network structure and other building blocks have fostered successful quality improvements. VCSQI has created a statewide database of 75,000 matched surgical and inpatient charge records dating from 2002 through 2011. The matched cost and quality data permits measurement of outcomes, resource use, and costs. The group's work also includes special studies, surveys, information sharing on practice patterns, workshops on data integrity, and in-depth review of outcomes and risk factors. By way of example, the majority of Virginia's heart programs adopted national guidelines and related protocols for intra-operative and post-operative blood use. Savings were achieved and patient outcomes improved as a result of coordinated efforts. However, the group is challenged to better synchronize efforts and minimize variations in how protocols are adopted. Full participation in specific quality initiatives may prove elusive since each program has a different set of priorities. While VCSQI has attained a self-supporting sustainability, garnering additional financial resources will augment its mission. Standardizing documentation on return on investment (ROI) and savings is a priority. Given that performance must be measured on a level playing field, rigorous data quality assurance needs to be emphasized. VCSQI's sustainability, recognized accomplishments, and manageable size can be replicated in other regions to achieve better patient care and improved cardiac surgical outcomes.

The Virginia Cardiac Surgery Quality Initiative

This is an overview of a statewide cardiac surgical consortium called the Virginia Cardiac Surgery Quality Initiative. Voluntary, self-funded, and not-for-profit, VCSQI is a collaboration of 17 hospitals and 13 cardiac surgical practices conducting virtually 100% of the open-heart surgical procedures in the Commonwealth of Virginia. The group uses a clinical/financial registry to help identify high-impact quality improvement (QI) processes benefiting cardiac surgery patients.

The VCSQI was initially convened in 1996 with the stated purpose to facilitate collaboration between hospitals and physicians in order to improve clinical quality across an entire state in programs of all sizes through data sharing, outcomes analysis, and process improvements. It was anticipated that a unified focus on quality would contain costs in cardiac surgical care by lowering complications, improving efficiency, and reducing resource utilization. Our database linking clinical and financial outcomes provides a means to set baseline measures and track changes.

In addition to a primary focus on quality, payment reform has been a central concern and priority of VCSQI. An unsolicited proposal was submitted in 2004 to the Center for Medicare and Medicaid Services (CMS) recommending a test of a global payment methodology for patients undergoing coronary bypass and valvular replacement/repair. This methodology also included financial incentives for the participating physicians if quality improvement targets were realized during the evaluation period. The methodology subsequently became the basis for the CMS Acute Care Episode (ACE) Demonstration for cardiac surgery and knee/hip replacements in Texas, Oklahoma, New Mexico, and Colorado. This demonstration remains in progress and should be completed on schedule.

VCSQI also worked with a major payer in the region to develop a pay-for-performance program aligning incentives for defined quality outcomes for hospitals and participating cardiac surgeons. This model was eventually applied to programs across the greater part of the country. Our clinical/financial data repository has additionally been used as a modeling tool to illustrate the financial impact of how improved clinical quality reduces inpatient costs and lowers post-operative complications and mortality. Besides outcome comparisons with the Society of Thoracic Surgeons (STS) National Cardiac Surgery Database, the group also benchmarks with indicators from the National Quality Forum (NQF) cardiac surgery quality measures, an indicator set that members of VCSQI helped establish.

VCSQI advocates for a locally-driven, tiered payment incentive with initial payments to surgeons and hospitals for participation in a clinical data registry. This is followed by payments for achieving or improving upon process and outcome measures. The premise is that sharing best-practice protocols across participating sites will result in fewer post-operative complications and improve use of resources because of more rapid diffusion of knowledge among trusted peers. A secondary outcome is better understanding of quality guided resource utilization management.

The primary focus remains improvement in quality outcomes in all patients undergoing cardiac surgical procedures in the Commonwealth of Virginia. The group has demonstrated that collaboration among all participants promotes regional accountability and can improve quality. VCSQI created an organizational structure and other building blocks that form a successful quality improvement network. Vigilant data quality assurance, use of leading technology, good documentation, proven methods, effective group processes, sound communications, and surgeon leadership are essential. Active ties with clinical staff in each heart program are important for fostering effective improvements.

VCSQI began and remains a truly multidisciplinary collaboration. Hospital members include two academic medical centers, two multi-hospital systems (one for-profit and one Catholic), two regionally integrated health systems plus a dozen regional medical centers and freestanding hospitals. Surgeons, nursing staff, perfusionists, administrators, clinical data managers, and other staff participate in both governance and clinical activities of the VCSQI.

Over the years, we have captured surgical performance and cost data on nearly 75,000 cases dating from 2002 through 2011. Quarterly and semi-annually, members upload files of de-identified, patient-level data for all adult cardiac surgery cases to a secure web site. We match clinical data from the STS adult cardiac surgery database with financial data from standardized hospital UB-04 files. Using these sources, Armus Corporation (San Mateo CA) developed the Outcomes3 database for VCSQI. Hospital-specific ratios (RCC) of cost-to-charges from Medicare Cost Reports are updated regularly to normalize hospital charges among participating hospitals. An application library, online report library, an *Annual Report*, and research activities are driven from the database. The online report library shows NQF cardiac surgical quality indicators for each member hospital along with state and national norms. There is also a chart library of operational indicators showing selected measures side-by-side for hospitals and trended forward from 2002.

VCSQI convenes meetings quarterly to discuss topics most relevant to members' concerns. Here is a sampling of representative recent meeting agenda items:

- Implementing an atrial fibrillation prevention prophylaxis;
- Adopting STS transfusion guidelines;
- Sharing insulin protocols and diabetes management strategies;
- Methods for reducing prolonged ventilation;
- Ways to promote early extubation;
- Predicting risk of acute kidney injury;
- Reducing deep sternal wound infections;
- Utilization of the internal mammary artery (IMA) in coronary artery bypass graft (CABG) procedures;
- Appropriate use of discharge medications;
- Determining the impact of Aprotinin usage on bleeding and risk;
- Identifying ways to reduce readmissions.

Group interactions have also included numerous special studies and surveys on practice patterns, annual workshops for data coordinators, and in-depth review of cardiac surgical risk assessment tools. A fast-track program for same day transfer from ICU to post operative step down units in CABG surgery has been assessed along with a variety of risk estimation models. Studies on the additive costs of post-operative complications have been conducted using an RCC-based costing method. Recently, VCSQI has affiliated nationally with data coordinators responsible for adult cardiac, congenital cardiac and general thoracic surgery registries in order to promote improved communication, consistency, and coordination for reporting outcomes in cardiac surgery.

Statewide Blood Use Protocol

As an example of one of our quality improvement initiatives, VCSQI adopted and promoted an opt-in blood utilization program following guideline from STS. (A video summary is available at: http://www.vcsqi.org/ blood_conservation.php.) On March 6, 2008, we convened a meeting on the topic of blood conservation in cardiac surgery. Surgeons from the University of Virginia Health System, the Inova Heart and Vascular Institute, and Virginia Commonwealth University's Pauley Heart Center (VCU) presented information on transfusion practices in Virginia and the proposed use of a red blood cell transfusion protocol. The event concluded with remarks from VCU's Dr. Bruce Spiess, one of the authors of the STS transfusion guidelines. As stated by his associate and head of VCU's cardiothoracic surgery program, Dr. Vigneshwar Kasirajan, "*The opportunity for a cooperative group of Centers of Excellence in cardiac surgery to prospectively evaluate transfusion will dramatically advance knowledge in this area.*"

Over the next two years, the majority of heart programs in Virginia implemented the protocol at different starting points and with some variations. We analyzed records for 14,259 patients from 2006 (pre-implementation) to 2010. Cases selected for study were all non-emergent, primary, isolated coronary artery bypass grafting operations. Patients were stratified according to whether the date of surgery was pre-guideline (n=7,059) or post-guideline (n=7,200). Differences in rates of major complications and risk-adjusted mortality were the primary surgical outcomes studied using multiple regression analysis.

Comparisons demonstrated significant reductions in the use of intra-operative and post-operative blood transfusion for participating programs. There were also associated declines in pneumonia, prolonged ventilation, renal failure, new onset hemodialysis, and the composite incidence of post-operative complications from the time at which the protocol was implemented. The incidence of operative mortality also declined. Further, the additive costs of cases forgoing transfusion were significantly lower than for transfused patients. The dramatic reduction in costs to health care providers and insurers by the reduction in complications as a result of such a transfusion protocol reportedly saved over $40 million dollars during the two-year term of the study. These results were presented as part of the first STS Webinar demonstrating quality improvement processes in March, 2012.

This coordinated, multi-site intervention illustrates the positive impact on outcomes that collaborative guideline implementation can have. However, challenges remain in synchronizing a group's efforts around quality initiatives, minimizing variations in how a protocol is adopted, as well as obtaining the consensus for full participation. Additional challenges relate to the ability to obtain financial resources which would improve documentation of workable benefits, as well as and limitations of such collaboration, and identify ways to promote staff buy-in.

An Integrated Perspective for Quality Improvement

VCSQI has approached performance improvement on a collaborative basis using an integrated perspective. The four components of our integrated model for improving quality include:

- *Outcomes Measurement* – Using outcomes indicators that are sensitive, actionable, and clinically relevant is a core activity in quality improvement. Selecting benchmarks that evolve as progress is achieved among top and lower quartile performers is desirable.
- *Data Quality Assurance* – Performance must be measured on a level playing field with rigorous data quality assurance. This can involve using IT-based rules, self-audits, workshops, monthly and quarterly communications, web-based forums, and mentoring to ensure data quality. Certification for data managers would be among several desirable end points.
- *Clinical Workflow Transformation* – Managing changes in workflow for clinical staff is a crucial element for improving outcomes in cardiac surgical care. Since the costs of cardiac surgery occur in a short interval, cost savings are highly correlated with improvements in outcomes.
- *Effective Communications* – Training, education, team development, and sharing of best practices are premised on frequent, structured, 'quality' exchanges among participants. Rapid access to data measuring the impact of a quality improvement initiative helps VCSQI's members make timely course corrections.

VCSQI uses a collaborative model to connect with participants, diffuse information rapidly, and synchronize interventions. VCSQI's Quality Committee has built its agenda around a set of quality indicators and clinical priorities.

Our ability to match cost and quality data permits measurement of the interactions between outcomes, resources used, and costs. A set of dashboards is available to track outcomes and progress. Measures are evaluated periodically with hospital-specific blinded, de-identified reports. These reports are circulated to all participants noting variances between best performers and under-performers. Individuals volunteer information on best practices that improve quality while others can adopt certain interventions. These practices can be scrutinized with medical outcomes literature and a methodology devised to guide data collection and detect statistically significant changes associated with an intervention. VCSQI rigorously protects members' confidential operational information to ensure its non-disclosure. However, some documentation is maintained on details of the interventions among participants.

Future Challenges

VCSQI is collaborative by design with an orientation toward innovation and performance improvement in cardiac surgery. Set in a competitive marketplace with continual leadership changes and external threats to viability, an organization of this nature is expected to encounter challenges. That said, the group has experienced a remarkable compatibility and a tendency to accommodate each other's differences rather than disintegrate.

VCSQI has created a work plan to remain relevant to its members. A focus on improving outcomes will continue to drive our agenda. In addition, better documentation on systems change efforts is needed along with more standardized savings methodologies and additional information to augment risk assessment.

Our technology partner, Armus Corporation, is continually testing ways to improve delivery of business intelligence to decision-makers. We intend to take advantage of web based distance learning resources to expose our model to organizations in different settings. Here are some resources and capacities that would make VCSQI an even stronger organization.

- *Improved Systems Change Documentation* – VCSQI's efforts to promote the adoption of best-practice protocols can be boosted with (1) more comprehensive on-site documentation of quality improvement efforts and (2) better use of webinars to convey information to broader audiences.
- *Adoption of Standardized Financial Reporting Methods* – In an effort to create more defensible study results, VCSQI is considering the adoption of CPA-certified financial reporting standards and actuarial methods to better compute savings and return on investment figures.
- *Risk Identification* – The group recognizes the importance of augmenting risk-adjusted STS data and cost measures with socio-economic indicators. Analysis will determine whether below average cardiac surgical outcomes are more prominent in rural, inner city, or low income clusters.
- *Delivery of Business Intelligence* – We want to improve delivery and reporting of specialized information to individuals leading change initiatives. Examining gaps between norms and actual performance can guide correction action plans. This process is aided with timely data.
- *Utilize Web-based Learning Tools* – VCSQI is experimenting with the delivery of content to more audiences with web-based social networking tools. The ability to facilitate webinars and use videoconferencing will broaden and enrich VCSQI's convening function.
- *Extend collaboration* – It would be opportune to take advantage of strong ties among surgeons in other states' cardiac surgical practices and with colleagues in cardiology to stimulate similar collaborative processes.

Attributes for Success

One of the best indicators of a successful collaboration is found in the 'tone' set by its leaders at a meeting. When there is a certain buzz in the air, one can recognize a healthy group. We believe that a professional environment that encourages open innovation improves probabilities of success. The presence of committed and energetic leaders who are highly regarded and listened to by the group is a key ingredient. Recognizing that surgery is a 'team sport', a multi-disciplinary team composition ensures sufficient depth, breadth, and balance. A manageable size and reasonably close proximity help with communications while a non-hierarchical structure may minimize conflicts. Moderate turnover is conducive to continuity. Competition between heart programs will always be a consideration.

A clear and concise mission statement can maximize buy-in by focusing on common interests. A group must see the need to make changes that positively impact patient health and reduce variations in outcomes across programs. Evidence of early and consistent 'wins' helps engage staff and reaffirm that there will be a favorable return-on-investment. It is vital that participants are not locked into specific initiatives and can address individual rather than collective priorities. Participants have to be willing to share information on strengths and weaknesses of the proposed data and adapt proven solutions to new and different circumstances. Trust and transparency are hallmarks of effective collaboration as is use of advanced technologies facilitating communications and analysis. It may help to use a neutral facilitator to motivate, solve problems, and foster trust. Of course, there is no substitute for an open and flexible process for identifying issues, reviewing evidence, comparing relative performance, and replicating best practices.

VCSQI considers its work far from complete. In many respects given national changes in delivery and payment, its work may just be beginning. The more things change, the more suited collaborative models are for sharing solutions. We recognize that there is still a need to provide information and learning opportunities to our peers. This is witnessed with the all-to-frequent e-mail messages saying, "*Does anyone out there have a blood conservation model they would be willing to share?*" Or, "*I've had difficulty recruiting physicians to participate in our cardiac initiative and learning network. While I'm working with our Medical Director to help with recruitment, do you have any suggestions?*"

MEMBER HOSPITALS AND SURGICAL PRACTICES

- Bon Secours Richmond Health System
    - St. Mary's Hospital
    - Memorial Regional Medical Center
- Bon Secours Heart Institute, Portsmouth
- Carilion Roanoke Memorial Hospital, Roanoke
- Centra Health (Lynchburg General Hospital), Lynchburg
- HCA
    - Levinson Heart Hospital at CJW Medical Center, Richmond
    - Henrico Doctor's Hospital, Richmond
    - Lewis-Gale Medical Center, Salem
- Inova Health System
    - Fairfax Hospital
    - Alexandria Hospital
- Mary Washington Hospital, Fredericksburg
- Riverside Regional Medical Center, Newport News
- Sentara Health System
    - Norfolk General Hospital
    - Virginia Beach General Hospital
- University of Virginia Health Sciences Center, Charlottesville
- Virginia Commonwealth University, Pauley Heart Center, Richmond
- Winchester Medical Center, Winchester

VCSQI PHYSICIAN MEMBERS

- Bon Secours Heart Institute, Portsmouth
- Cardiac Surgery Specialists, Richmond
- Cardiothoracic Surgery Associates, Falls Church

- Cardiac and Thoracic Surgical Associates, Richmond
- Carilion Cardiothoracic Surgery, Roanoke
- Centra Health Cardiothoracic Surgery, Lynchburg
- Medical College of Virginia Physician Practice, Richmond
- Mid-Atlantic Cardiothoracic Surgery, Norfolk
- Roanoke Valley Cardiovascular Surgery, Salem
- Tidewater Cardiothoracic, Newport News
- University of Virginia Health System, Charlottesville
- Valley Health Cardiothoracic & Vascular Surgeons, Winchester
- VCS, Inc., Fredericksburg

REFERENCES

[1] la Par, D. J., Ailawadi, G., Bhamidipati, C. M., Stukenborg, G. J., Crosby, I. K., Kern, J. A., Kron, I. L. Small Prosthesis Size in Aortic Valve Replacement Does Not Affect Mortality. *Ann Thorac Surg* 2011. (In press).

[2] Gazoni, Leo M., Speir, Alan M., Irving, Kron L., Fonner, Clifford, Crosby, Ivan K. Elective Thoracic Aortic Aneurysm Surgery: Better Outcomes from High-Volume Centers. *JACS*, 2010, 210(5): 855-860.

[3] la Par, Damien, Hennessy, Sara, Fonner, Eddie, Kern, John, Irving Kron, Ailawadi, Gorav. Does Urgent or Emergent Status Influence Choice in Mitral Valve Operations? An Analysis of Outcomes from the Virginia Cardiac Surgery Quality Initiative. *Annals of Thoracic Surgery*, 2010; 90:153-160.

[4] Speir, Alan M., Rich, Jeffrey B., Crosby, Ivan, Fonner, Edwin, Jr. Regional Collaboration as a Model for Fostering Accountability and Transforming Healthcare. *Seminars in Thoracic and Cardiovascular Surgery* 2009: 21:12-19.

[5] Speir, Alan M., Kasirajan, Vigneshwar, Barnett, Scott D. and Fonner, Edwin, Jr. Additive Cost of Postoperative Complications for Isolated Coronary Artery Bypass Grafting Patients in Virginia. *Annals of Thoracic Surgery* 2009; 88: 40-46. Presented at the 45th annual meeting of the Society of Thoracic Surgeons, San Francisco CA, January 2009.

[6] Rich, Jeffrey B., Speir, Alan M, Fonner, Edwin, Jr. Making a Business Case for Quality by Regional Information Sharing Involving Cardiothoracic Surgery. *The American Heart Hospital Journal*, 4, no. 2 (Spring 2006): 142-147.

[7] Bhamidipati, Castigliano M., la Par, Damien J., Fonner, Edwin Jr., Kern, John A., Kron, Irving L., Ailawadi, Gorav. Outcomes and Cost of Cardiac Surgery in Octogenarians is Related to Type of Operation: *A Multi-Institutional Analysis.* 2010 ACC Meeting, Atlanta GA.

[8] Fonner, Edwin Jr., Kasirajan, Vigneshwar, Speir, Alan M., and Clifford Edwin Fonner. Ethnicity and Cost Following Isolated Coronary Artery Bypass Surgery: *Results from the Virginia Cardiac Surgery Quality Initiative.* Poster presented at the Academy Health Annual Research Meeting, Chicago IL, June 28-30, 2009.

[9] Fonner, Edwin Jr., Vigneshwar Kasirajan, Speir Alan M., and Clifford Edwin Fonner. *Measuring Changes in Care Practices and Postoperative Outcomes by Ethnicity and Gender Using a Disease Registry by a Cardiac Surgery Quality Improvement*

Consortium. Poster presented at the Academy Health Annual Research Meeting, Chicago IL, June 28-30, 2009.

[10] Speir, Alan M., and Edwin Fonner, Jr. *Costs of Postoperative Complications in Cardiac Surgery*. Poster presented at the Cleveland Clinic Foundation, Orthopaedic and Rheumatology Care Quality Innovation Summit, Cleveland OH, May 13-15, 2009.

[11] Speir, Alan M., and Edwin Fonner, Jr. *A Model for Relating P4P to CQI*. Poster presented at the Cleveland Clinic Foundation, Orthopaedic and Rheumatology Care Quality Innovation Summit, Cleveland OH, May 13-15, 2009.

[12] Speir, Alan M., and Edwin Fonner, Jr. *A Multidisciplinary, Regional, Evidence-based QI Collaboration in Virginia*. Poster presented at the Cleveland Clinic Foundation, Orthopaedic and Rheumatology Care Quality Innovation Summit, Cleveland OH, May 13-15, 2009.

[13] Speir, Alan M, Barnett, Scott, Smith, Judy, and Edwin Fonner, Jr. Gender Differences in Outcomes Following On-pump CABG and Off-pump CABG: *Results from the Virginia Cardiac Surgery Quality Initiative Registry*. Poster presented at the America Heart Association Quality of care and Outcomes Research in Cardiovascular Disease and Stroke Conference, Washington DC, April 23-25, 2009.

[14] Speir, Alan M., Vigneshwar, Kasirajan, Barnett, Scott D. and Edwin Fonner, Jr. The Association of Gender and Age on Cost Following Isolated Coronary Artery Bypass Surgery: *Results from the Virginia Cardiac Surgery Quality Initiative*. Poster presented at the America Heart Association Quality of care and Outcomes Research in Cardiovascular Disease and Stroke Conference, Washington DC, April 23-25, 2009.

[15] Barnett, Scott, Fonner, Ed, Rich, Jeff, and Alan Speir. Summary of Results of the Virginia Cardiac Surgery Quality Initiative: Valve Replacement Costs and Mortality. Poster at the Academy Health Annual Research meeting, Seattle WA, June 25-27, 2006.

[16] la Par, D. J., Mulloy, D. P., Stone, M. L., Crosby, I. K., Lau, C. L., Kron, I. L., and G. Ailawadi. *Concomitant Tricuspid Valve Surgery Affects Outcomes Following Mitral Operations: A multi-institutional, statewide analysis*. Southern Thoracic Surgical Association (STSA), 58th Annual Meeting. November 11, 2011. San Antonio, TX.

[17] la Par, D. J., Mulloy, D. P., Crosby, I. K., Lim, D. S., Kern, J. A., Kron, I. L., and G. Ailawadi. *Contemporary Outcomes for Surgical Mitral Valve Repair: A Benchmark for Evaluating Emerging Mitral Valve Technology*. 2011 Mitral Conclave, American Association for Thoracic Surgery. May 6, 2011. New York, NY.

[18] la Par, D. J., Ailawadi, G., Bhamidipati, C. M., Stukenborg, G. J., Crosby, I. K., Kern, J. A., and I.L. Kron. *Small Prosthesis Size in Aortic Valve Replacement Does Not Affect Mortality*. 47th Annual Meeting of the Society of Thoracic Surgeons. February 1, 2011. San Diego, CA.

[19] Speir, Alan M. *AMA Pathways to Success: What physicians need to know about ACOs and the coming revolution in payment practices*. Specialist and primary care strategies for improving quality and lowering costs, Raleigh, NC, July 16, 2011.

[20] Speir, Alan M. AMA Payment Pathways Seminar: *2011 Joint Surgical Advocacy Conference - How Surgeons Can Lead the Value-Based Payment Transformation*, Washington, DC, March 28, 2011.

[21] Fonner, Edwin, Jr. *Overview of VCSQI* at the Kansas/Missouri Regional Data Managers Meeting, Kansas City KS, October 29, 2010.

[22] Fonner, Edwin, Jr. *Overview of VCSQI* at the Texas Regional Data Managers Meeting, San Antonio TX, September 10, 2010.
[23] Speir, Alan M. Physicians Leading Through Change – AMA Presidents Forum, *AMA Annual Meeting*, Washington, DC, March 9, 2009.
[24] Fonner, Edwin, Jr. *Sutter Health's Quarterly Cardiac Surgery Quality Meeting,* Lafayette CA, June 2009. Quality Improvement Initiatives with the Virginia Cardiac Surgery Quality Initiative.
[25] Fonner, Edwin, Jr. *The Virginia Cardiac Surgery Quality Initiative: A Regional QI Program.* Keynote address at the 13th Annual Statewide Meeting, Clinical Outcomes Assessment Program (COAP), Seattle WA, May 19, 2009.
[26] Fonner, Edwin, Jr. The Virginia Cardiac Quality Improvement Project. Presented at the *The Future of Provider-Led Database Systems in Medicine' symposium*, UNC Chapel Hill, September 19, 2006.

In: Quality Improvement
Editors: K. W. Lobdell and S. C. Stamou
ISBN: 978-1-62417-390-5

Chapter 10

Collaboration in Cardiac Surgical Quality Improvement: The Michigan Experience

Tad Boeve**, Rich Prager and Patty Theurer
Michigan Society of Thoracic and Cardiovascular Surgeons Quality Collaborative,
East Lansing, MI, US

Abstract

The Michigan Society of Thoracic and Cardiovascular Surgeons (MSTCVS) Quality Collaborative is a unique regional collaborative of physicians, hospitals and the largest private insurer in Michigan designed to improve the quality of care delivered to all patients in Michigan undergoing cardiac surgery. All cardiac surgery sites in Michigan participate in the Society of Thoracic Surgeons (STS) database and in the quality collaborative. In 2005 Blue Cross Blue Shield (BCBS) of Michigan began to partially fund the cardiac-surgeon led quality collaborative. The collaborative holds quarterly meetings where selected performance measures from all programs are reviewed and compared. Reviewing our collaborative data revealed a fairly wide distribution of results, especially in the earlier years. Sharing results and "best practices" has allowed many programs to improve their performance in selected measures When all sites participate in a voluntary fashion, learning can occur across typical competitive barriers and a "learning community" created. The lessons learned from one site can be applied at a different site. The MSTCVS Quality Collaborative has accomplished a major milestone in elevating the collective performance of the entire state of Michigan to the upper echelon of national ranks. During our earlier reporting periods (2006 and 2007) the collective performance of the Michigan sites when compared to the nation as a whole was not distinguishable. In our later reporting (2010-2011) Michigan as a whole achieved a 3 star rating from the Society of Thoracic Surgeons, demonstrating that within 99% probability we were performing approximately in the top decile of performance. The MSTCVS Quality Collaborative has translated an interest in improving quality of care into demonstrated benefit for the patients in our state. While much work remains to be done there is much to

---

* Email for corresponding author: Boeve@wmcts.com, Theodore J. Boeve MD FACS, West Michigan Cardiothoracic Surgeons.

be said for regional collaboration with focus on site specific goals to improve quality of care.

The Society of Thoracic Surgeons
Adult Cardiac Surgery Database
Data Collection Form Version 2.73
January 14, 2011

D. Risk Factors

Weight (kg): ________ | Height (cm): ________

Cigarette Smoker: ☐ Yes ☐ No (If Yes →) Current Cigarette Smoker: ☐ Yes ☐ No
Other Tobacco Use: ☐ Yes ☐ No

Family History of Premature Coronary Artery Disease: ☐ Yes ☐ No | Last Hematocrit: ________ | Last WBC Count: ________

Platelet Count Prior to Surgery: ______ | International Normalized Ratio prior to Surgery: ________

HIT Antibodies ☐ Yes ☐ No ☐ Not Applicable | Total Bilirubin Prior to Surgery:

Total Albumin Prior to Surgery: ______ | A1c Level prior to surgery: ______ | Last Creatinine Level Prior to Surgery: ______

Diabetes: ☐ Yes ☐ No (If Yes →) Diabetes-Control: ☐ None ☐ Diet ☐ Oral ☐ Insulin ☐ Other

Dyslipidemia: ☐ Yes ☐ No | Dialysis: ☐ Yes ☐ No | MELD Score: ______ (System Calculation) | Hypertension: ☐ Yes ☐ No

Infectious Endocarditis: ☐ Yes ☐ No
(If Yes →) Infectious Endocarditis Type: ☐ Treated ☐ Active
Infectious Endocarditis Culture:
☐ Culture negative ☐ Staphylococcus aureus ☐ Streptococcus species
☐ Coagulase negative staphylococcus ☐ Enterococcus species ☐ Fungal ☐ Other

Chronic Lung Disease: ☐ No ☐ Mild ☐ Moderate ☐ Severe

Pulmonary Function Test Done: ☐ Yes ☐ No
(If Yes →) FEV1 % Predicted: ________
DLCO Test Performed: ☐ Yes ☐ No (If Yes →) DLCO % Predicted: _____

Arterial Blood Gas Performed: ☐ Yes ☐ No (If Yes →) Oxygen Level: ________ Carbon Dioxide Level: ________

Home Oxygen: ☐ Yes ☐ No | Inhaled Medication or Oral Bronchodilator Therapy: ☐ Yes ☐ No
Sleep Apnea: ☐ Yes ☐ No | Liver Disease: ☐ Yes ☐ No
Immunocompromise Present: ☐ Yes ☐ No | Peripheral Artery Disease: ☐ Yes ☐ No
Unresponsive Neurologic State: ☐ Yes ☐ No | Syncope: ☐ Yes ☐ No

Cerebrovascular Disease: ☐ Yes ☐ No
(If Yes →) Prior CVA: ☐ Yes ☐ No (If Yes →) Prior CVA-When: ☐ Recent (<=2 wk.) ☐ Remote (>2 wk.)
CVD TIA: ☐ Yes ☐ No
CVD Carotid stenosis: ☐ None ☐ Right ☐ Left ☐ Both
(If "Right" or "Both" →) Severity of stenosis on the right carotid artery: ☐ 80 - 99% ☐ 100%
History of previous carotid artery surgery and/or stenting: ☐ Yes ☐ No

Illicit Drug Use: ☐ Yes ☐ No | Alcohol Use: ☐ <=1 drink/week ☐ 2-7 drinks/week ☐ >=8 drinks/week

Pneumonia: ☐ No ☐ Recent ☐ Remote | Mediastinal Radiation: ☐ Yes ☐ No | Cancer Within 5 Years: ☐ Yes ☐ No

Five Meter Walk Test Done: ☐ Yes ☐ No
(If Yes →) Time 1: ______ (secs) Time 2: ______ (secs) Time 3: ______ (secs)

F. Preoperative Cardiac Status

Prior Myocardial Infarction: ☐ Yes ☐ No (If Yes ↓)
MI When: ☐ <=6 Hrs ☐ >6 Hrs but <24 Hrs ☐ 1 to 7 Days ☐ 8 to 21 Days ☐ >21 Days

Anginal Classification Within 2 weeks: ☐ No Symptoms, No Angina ☐ CCA I ☐ CCA II ☐ CCA III ☐ CCA IV

Heart Failure Within 2 weeks: Classification-NYHA: ☐ Class I ☐ Class II ☐ Class III ☐ Class IV
☐ Yes ☐ No (If Yes →)

Prior Heart failure: ☐ Yes ☐ No

Cardiac Presentation on Admission: ☐ No Symptoms, No Angina ☐ Symptoms Unlikely to be Ischemia ☐ Stable Angina ☐ Unstable Angina ☐ Non-ST Elevation MI (Non-STEMI) ☐ ST Elevation MI (STEMI)

Cardiogenic Shock: ☐ Yes ☐ No

Resuscitation: ☐ Yes ☐ No

Arrhythmia When: ☐ None ☐ Remote ☐ Recent (If Recent ↓)
Arrhythmia Type: Vtach/Vfib: ☐ Yes ☐ No | Second Degree Heart Block: ☐ Yes ☐ No
Sick Sinus Syndrome: ☐ Yes ☐ No | Third Degree Heart Block: ☐ Yes ☐ No
Afib/Aflutter: ☐ Yes ☐ No
(If Yes →) **Type:** ☐ Paroxysmal ☐ Continuous/Persistent

Figure 1. a.

G. Preoperative Medications

Beta Blockers: ☐ Yes ☐ No ☐ Contraindicated

ACE or ARB Inhibitors Within 48 Hours: ☐ Yes ☐ No

Nitrates-I.V.: ☐ Yes ☐ No

Anticoagulants: ☐ Yes ☐ No (If Yes→) Medication Name: ☐ Heparin (Unfractionated) ☐ Heparin (Low Molecular) ☐ Thrombin Inhibitors ☐ Other

Preoperative Antiarrhythmics: ☐ Yes ☐ No

Coumadin: ☐ Yes ☐ No

Inotropes: ☐ Yes ☐ No

Steroids: ☐ Yes ☐ No

Aspirin: ☐ Yes ☐ No

Lipid Lowering: ☐ Yes ☐ No (If Yes→) Medication Type: ☐ Statin ☐ Non-statin ☐ Both

ADP Inhibitors Within Five Days: ☐ Yes ☐ No (If Yes→) ADP Inhibitors Discontinuation: _______ Days

Antiplatelets Within 5 Days: ☐ Yes ☐ No

Glycoprotein IIb/IIIa Inhibitor: ☐ Yes ☐ No (Medication: ☐ Abciximab (ReoPro) ☐ Eptifibatide ☐ Tirofiban (Aggrastat)

Thrombolytics within 48 hours: ☐ Yes ☐ No

H. Hemodynamics/Cath/Echo

Cardiac Catheterization Performed: ☐ Yes ☐ No (If Yes→) Cardiac Catheterization Date: __ __/__ __/__ __ __ __

Number Diseased Vessels: ☐ None ☐ One ☐ Two ☐ Three

Left Main Disease >= 50%: ☐ Yes ☐ No

Proximal LAD >= 70%: ☐ Yes ☐ No

Ejection Fraction Done: ☐ Yes ☐ No (If Yes ↓)

Ejection Fraction: _________ (%)

Ejection Fraction Method: ☐ LV Gram ☐ Radionucleotide ☐ Estimate ☐ ECHO ☐ MRI/CT ☐ Other

LV Systolic Dimension: (mm) | LV End-Diastolic Dimension: (mm)

PA Systolic Pressure Measured: ☐ Yes ☐ No PA Systolic Pressure: _______ mmHg(highest prior to surgery)

J. Coronary Bypass

(If OpCAB = Yes ↓)

Hybrid Procedure CAB and PCI Performed: ☐ Yes ☐ No (If Yes ↓)

Status: ☐ Planned - concurrent ☐ Planned - staged ☐ Unplanned

PCI Procedure Performed: ☐ Angioplasty ☐ Stent

Number of Distal Anastomoses with Arterial Conduits: _______

Number of Distal Anastomoses with Venous Conduits: _______ (If>0 ↓)

Vein Harvest Technique: ☐ Endoscopic ☐ Direct Vision (open) ☐ Both ☐ Cryopreserved

(If "Endoscopic", "Direct Vision (open)" or "Both"→) Saphenous Vein Harvest Time: ________ (minutes)

Saphenous Vein Preparation Time: ________ (minutes)

Internal Mammary Artery used for Grafts: ☐ Left IMA ☐ Right IMA ☐ Both IMAs ☐ No IMA

(If No IMA→) Indicate Primary Reason: ☐ The IMA is not a suitable conduit due to size or flow ☐ Subclavian stenosis ☐ Previous cardiac or thoracic surgery ☐ Previous mediastinal radiation ☐ Emergent or salvage procedure ☐ No LAD disease

(If Left, Right or Both IMAs →) Total # of Distal Anastomoses done using IMA grafts: ________

IMA Harvest Technique: ☐ Direct Vision (open) ☐ Thoracoscopy ☐ Combination ☐ Robotic Assist

Number of Radial Arteries Used for Grafts: __________ (If >0 ↓)

Number of Radial Artery Distal Anastomoses: _________

Radial Distal Anastomoses Harvest Technique: ☐ Endoscopic ☐ Direct Vision (open) ☐ Both

Radial Artery Harvest Time: __________ (minutes)

Radial Artery Preparation Time: __________ (minutes)

Number Other Arterial Distal Anastomoses Used (other than radial or IMA): ________

1 = Left Main	4 = Distal LAD	7 = Circumflex	10 = OM 3	13 = PLB
2 = Prox LAD	5 = Diagonal 1	8 = OM 1	11 = RCA	14 = AM branches
3 = Mid LAD	6 = Diagonal 2	9 = OM 2	12 = PDA	15 = Ramus

		1	2	3	4	5	6	7	8	9	10
	CABG NUMBER	1	2	3	4	5	6	7	8	9	10
GRAFT DONE	Yes	N									
	No	A									

Figure 1. b.

O. Post Operative

Postoperative Creatinine Level: ____________

Blood Products Used Postoperatively: ☐ Yes ☐ No (If Yes ↓)

Red Blood Cell Units: ______ Fresh Frozen Plasma Units: ______ Cryoprecipitate Units: ______ Platelet Units: ______

Extubated in OR: ☐ Yes ☐ No

Re-intubated During Hospital Stay: ☐ Yes ☐ No (If yes →) Additional Hours Ventilated: ______

ICU Visit: ☐ Yes ☐ No (If Yes →) Initial ICU Hours: ______

Readmission to ICU: ☐ Yes ☐ No (If Yes →) Additional ICU Hours: ________

Post Op Echo Performed: ☐ Yes ☐ No (If Yes ↓)

Highest level aortic insufficiency found: ☐ None ☐ Trace/trivial ☐ Mild ☐ Moderate ☐ Severe

Highest level mitral insufficiency found: ☐ None ☐ Trace/trivial ☐ Mild ☐ Moderate ☐ Severe

Highest level tricuspid insufficiency found: ☐ None ☐ Trace/trivial ☐ Mild ☐ Moderate ☐ Severe

Post Op Ejection Fraction Done: ☐ Yes ☐ No (If Yes ↓)

Post Op Ejection Fraction: ______ (%)

Cardiac Enzymes (biomarkers) Drawn: ☐ Yes ☐ No (If Yes →) Peak CKMB: ______ Peak Troponin I ______ Peak Troponin T ______

12-Lead EKG Findings: ☐ Not performed ☐ No significant changes ☐ New Pathological Q-wave or LBBB

Imaging Study Findings:

☐ Not performed

☐ Angiographic evidence of new thrombosis or occlusion of graft or native coronary

☐ Imaging evidence of new loss of viable myocardium

☐ No evidence of new myocardial injury

P. Postoperative Events

In Hospital Postoperative Event Occurred: ☐ Yes ☐ No (If Yes ↓)

Operative

ReOp for Bleeding /Tamponade: ☐ Yes ☐ No (If Yes →) Bleed Timing: ☐ Acute ☐ Late

ReOp for Valvular Dysfunction: ☐ Yes ☐ No

ReOp for Graft Occlusion: ☐ Yes ☐ No

ReOp for Other Cardiac Reasons: ☐ Yes ☐ No

ReOp for Other Non-Cardiac Reasons: ☐ Yes ☐ No

Open chest with planned delayed sternal closure: ☐ Yes ☐ No

Sternotomy Issue: ☐ Yes ☐ No (If Yes →) Sternal instability/dehiscence (sterile): ☐ Yes ☐ No

Infection (see CDC definitions in training manual)

Surgical Site Infection: ☐ Yes ☐ No (If Yes ↓)

Sternal Superficial Wound Infection: ☐ Yes ☐ No

Deep Sternal Infection: ☐ Yes ☐ No

Mediastinitis: ☐ Yes ☐ No (If Yes ↓)

Diagnosis Date: __ __/__ __/__ __ __ __ (mm/dd/yyyy)

Secondary Procedure Open with Packing/Irrigation: ☐ Yes ☐ No

Secondary Procedure Wound Vac: ☐ Yes ☐ No

Secondary Procedure Muscle Flap: ☐ Yes ☐ No

Secondary Procedure Omental Flap: ☐ Yes ☐ No

Thoracotomy: ☐ Yes ☐ No

Conduit Harvest or Cannulation Site: ☐ Yes ☐ No

Wound Intervention - Open with Packing/Irrigation: ☐ Yes ☐ No

Wound Intervention - Wound Vac - ☐ Yes ☐ No

Sepsis: ☐ Yes ☐ No (If Yes →) Positive Blood Cultures: ☐ Yes ☐ No

Neurologic

Postoperative Stroke (Perm>24 hours): ☐ Yes ☐ No

Transient Ischemic Attack (TIA): ☐ Yes ☐ No

Encephalopathy: ☐ None ☐ Anoxic ☐ Embolic ☐ Drug ☐ Metabolic ☐ Intracranial Bleeding ☐ Other

Paralysis: ☐ Yes ☐ No (If Yes →) Paralysis Type: ☐ Transient ☐ Permanent

Pulmonary

Prolonged Ventilation: ☐ Yes ☐ No   Pneumonia: ☐ Yes ☐ No

Venous Thromboembolism - VTE: ☐ Yes ☐ No (If Yes ↓)

Pulmonary Thromboembolism: ☐ Yes ☐ No   Deep Venous Thrombosis: ☐ Yes ☐ No

Pleural Effusion Requiring Drainage: ☐ Yes ☐ No

Renal

Renal Failure: ☐ Yes ☐ No } (If Yes ↓)

Dialysis (Newly Required): ☐ Yes ☐ No (If Yes →) Required after Hospital Discharge: ☐ Yes ☐ No

Ultra Filtration Required: ☐ Yes ☐ No

Vascular

Iliac/Femoral Dissection: ☐ Yes ☐ No   Acute Limb Ischemia: ☐ Yes ☐ No

Other

Rhythm Disturbance Requiring Permanent Device: ☐ Pacemaker ☐ ICD ☐ Pacemaker/ICD ☐ None

Cardiac Arrest: ☐ Yes ☐ No   Anticoagulant Event: ☐ Yes ☐ No

Tamponade (Non-Surgical Intervention): ☐ Yes ☐ No   Gastro-Intestinal Event: ☐ Yes ☐ No

Multi-System Failure: ☐ Yes ☐ No   Atrial Fibrillation: ☐ Yes ☐ No

Aortic Dissection: ☐ Yes ☐ No   Recurrent Laryngeal Nerve Injury: ☐ Yes ☐ No

Phrenic Nerve Injury: ☐ Yes ☐ No   Other: ☐ Yes ☐ No

Figure 1. c.

Q. Mortality

Mortality: ☐ Yes ☐ No	Discharge Status: ☐ Alive ☐ Dead	Status at 30 days After Surgery: ☐ Alive ☐ Dead ☐ Unknown

Primary method used to verify 30-day status:
☐ Phone call to patient or family ☐ Evidence of life in medical record ☐ Social Security Death Master File
☐ Letter from medical provider ☐ Office visit to surgeon >= 30 days after procedure ☐ Other

(If Mortality = Yes ↓)
Operative Death: ☐ Yes ☐ No
Mortality - Date __ __/__ __/__ __ __ __ (mm/dd/yyyy)
Location of Death: ☐ OR During Initial Surgery ☐ Hospital (Other than OR) ☐ Home ☐ Extended Care Facility ☐ Hospice ☐ Acute Rehabilitation ☐ OR During Reoperation ☐ Unknown ☐ Other
Primary Cause of Death (select only one)
☐ Cardiac ☐ Neurologic ☐ Renal ☐ Vascular ☐ Infection ☐ Pulmonary ☐ Valvular ☐ Unknown ☐ Other

R. Discharge

(If Discharge Status = Alive ↓)

ADP Inhibitors:	☐ Yes ☐ No
Antiarrhythmics:	☐ Yes ☐ No
Aspirin:	☐ Yes ☐ No ☐ Contraindicated
ACE or ARB Inhibitors:	☐ Yes ☐ No, contraindicated ☐ No, not indicated
Beta Blockers:	☐ Yes ☐ No ☐ Contraindicated
Lipid Lowering:	☐ Yes ☐ No ☐ Contraindicated (If Yes →) ☐ Statin ☐ Non Statin ☐ Both ☐ Other
Coumadin:	☐ Yes ☐ No
Direct Thrombin Inhibitors:	☐ Yes ☐ No
Discharge Location:	☐ Home ☐ Extended Care/Transitional Care Unit/Rehab ☐ Other Hospital ☐ Nursing Home ☐ Hospice ☐Other
Cardiac Rehabilitation Referral:	☐ Yes ☐ No ☐ Not Applicable
Smoking Cessation Counseling:	☐ Yes ☐ No ☐ Not Applicable

S. Readmission

(If Discharge Status = Alive ↓)

Readmit <=30 Days from Date of Procedure: ☐ Yes ☐ No (If Yes ↓)

Readmit Primary Reason:
- ☐ Anticoagulation Complication - Valvular
- ☐ Anticoagulation Complication - Pharmacological
- ☐ Arrhythmia/Heart Block
- ☐ Congestive Heart Failure
- ☐ Myocardial Infarction and/or Recurrent Angina
- ☐ Pericardial Effusion and/or Tamponade
- ☐ Pneumonia or other Respiratory Complication
- ☐ Coronary Artery Dysfunction
- ☐ Valve Dysfunction
- ☐ Infection - Deep Sternum / Mediastinitis
- ☐ Infection - Conduit Harvest Site
- ☐ Renal Failure
- ☐ TIA
- ☐ Permanent CVA
- ☐ Acute Vascular Complication
- ☐ Subacute Endocarditis
- ☐ VAD Complication
- ☐ Transplant Rejection
- ☐ PE
- ☐ DVT
- ☐ Other - Related Readmission
- ☐ Other - Nonrelated Readmission

Readmit Primary Procedure:
- ☐ OR for Bleeding
- ☐ Pacemaker Insertion / AICD
- ☐ PCI
- ☐ Pericardiotomy / Pericardiocentesis
- ☐ OR for Coronary Arteries
- ☐ OR for Valve
- ☐ OR for Sternal Debridement / Muscle Flap
- ☐ Dialysis
- ☐ OR for Vascular
- ☐ No Procedure Performed
- ☐ Other Procedure
- ☐ Unknown

Figure 1. d.

Figure 1. a-d. This figure demonstrates a portion of the data collected for the STS database for each patient undergoing cardiac surgery.

The Michigan Society of Thoracic and Cardiovascular Surgeons (MSTCVS) Quality Collaborative is a unique regional collaborative of physicians, hospitals and the largest private insurer in Michigan designed to improve the quality of care delivered to all patients in Michigan undergoing cardiac surgery. The collaborative has its roots in the history and success of the MSTCVS. The MSTCVS originated in 1965 as the Michigan Society of Thoracic Surgeons with Dr. Cameron Haight as the first President. 17 of the 60 board certified thoracic surgeons attended the first meeting. Since 1965 the society has met annually and grown in numbers and scope of influence. A tradition of holding the annual meeting in the summer at a family friendly resort in Northern Michigan developed. The scientific format was enhanced by inviting nationally prominent speakers, adding specific lectures and eventually a resident scientific paper competition. [1] Entertainment for members and their families as well as product vendors was always included. The summer meeting became increasingly popular and the state society membership grew steadily. Personal and professional relationships grew across the state. In 2002 the society recognized a unique opportunity to examine cardiac surgical outcomes in an attempt to provide the best and most uniform care possible across the state. In addition, the Society believed its members had a professional responsibility to build a forum and platform to demonstrate results and safety to the major insurers and employers in our state. Membership expanded voluntarily to include each of the 33 sites performing cardiac surgery in Michigan. Each site also initiated or continued participation in the Society of Thoracic Surgeons Adult Database (STS). The STS database is the cornerstone for outcomes and surgical benchmarking for the cardiac surgery community.

Cardiac surgeons have long recognized their responsibility to record results and work toward continued improvement in their surgical outcomes. The STS National Database was established in 1989 as an initiative for quality improvement and patient safety among cardiothoracic surgeons. Participation is voluntary and requires considerable time and effort to collect accurate data. The database contains patient demographic data, technical details of the operation performed, and detailed 30 day outcome measures. The Adult Cardiac Surgery Database contains more than 4.5 million surgical records and represents an estimated 94 percent of all adult cardiac surgery centers across the U. S. [2] The database allows any participating site to measure their risk-adjusted results against other like-sized programs and against national averages. See Figure 1 (a-d).

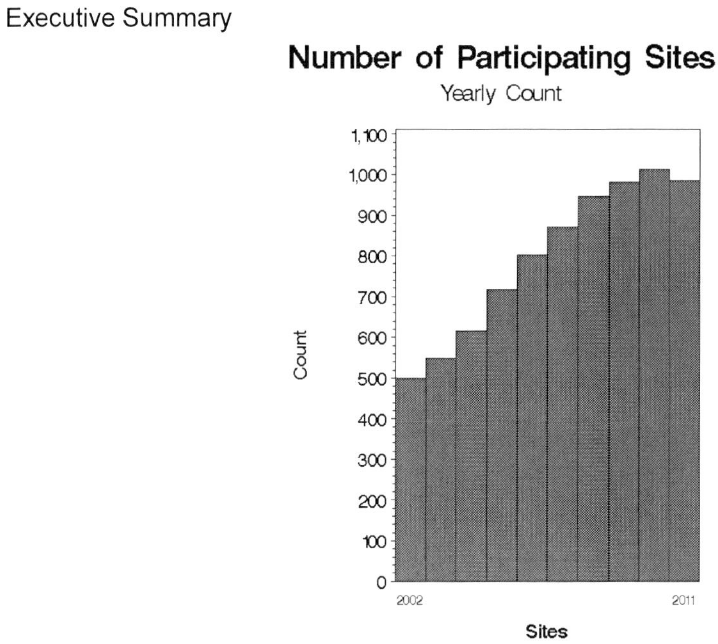

Figure 2. This figure demonstrates the number of programs submitting data to the STS database.

Each site that participates in this database inputs data on each patient and receives bi annual reports of their site-specific observed and expected results for each particular major procedure performed. The STS has developed robust risk adjustment algorithms to allow detailed expected results based on the patient population in its database as well as composite metrics for isolated coronary bypass procedures and isolated aortic valve procedures. [3] Periodically the risk adjustment calculations are adjusted to keep them current with year to year results. This database is a powerful tool for stratifying program results and identifying areas for site specific results. There are over 1050 sites participating in the adult database yielding over 1.5 million cumulative coronary artery bypass (CAB) procedures in the database, Figure 2 and 3. One can also see the steady decline in coronary artery bypass mortality demonstrated during the time of database use. See Figure 4. Figure 5 demonstrates the performance of a typical participating site in graphical form with regard to CAB mortality.

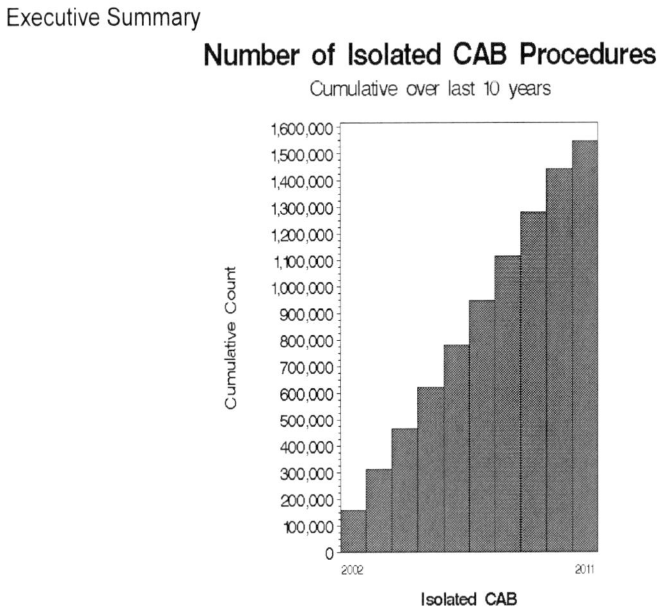

Figure 3. This figure demonstrates the cumulative number of coronary artery bypass procedures in the database.

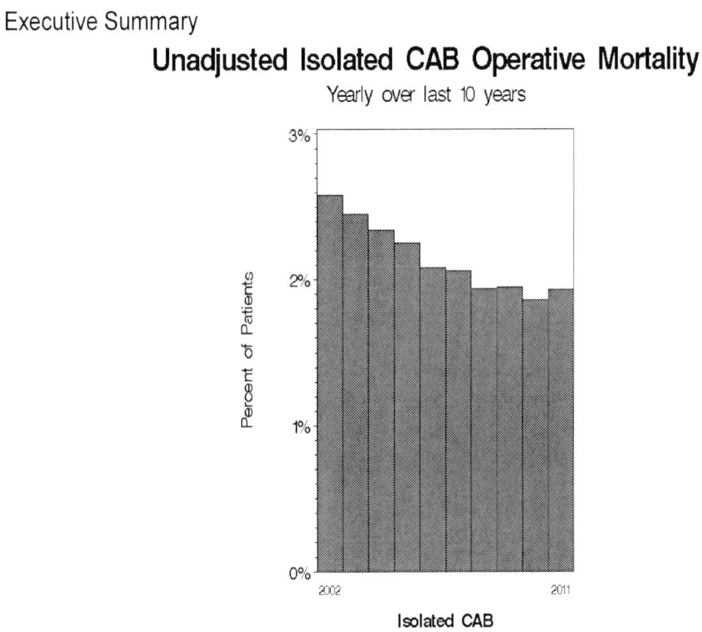

Figure 4. This figure demonstrates the decrease in coronary artery bypass mortality over time.

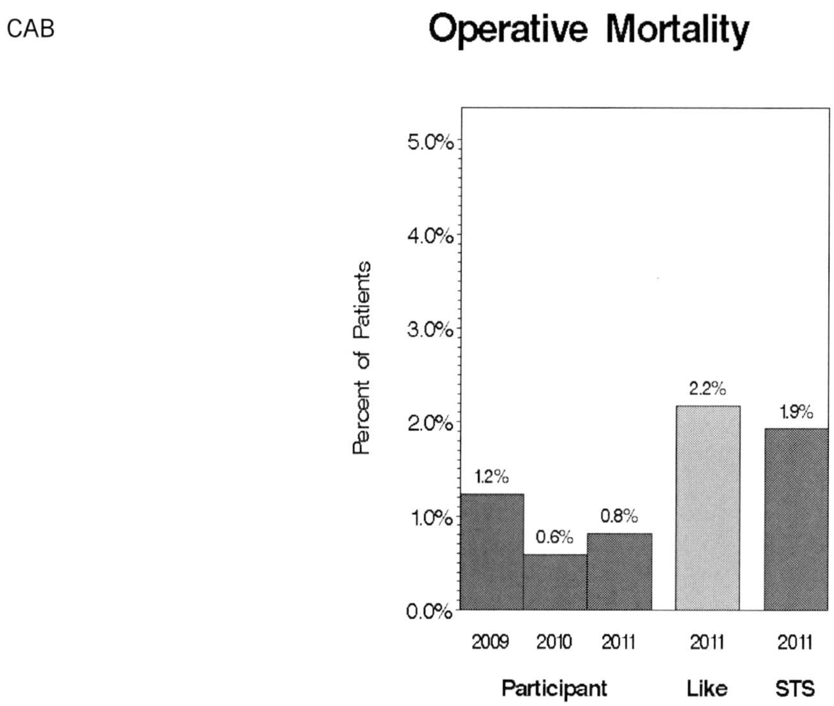

Figure 5. This figure demonstrates the performance of a typical program compared to other like- sized programs and compared to the STS average.

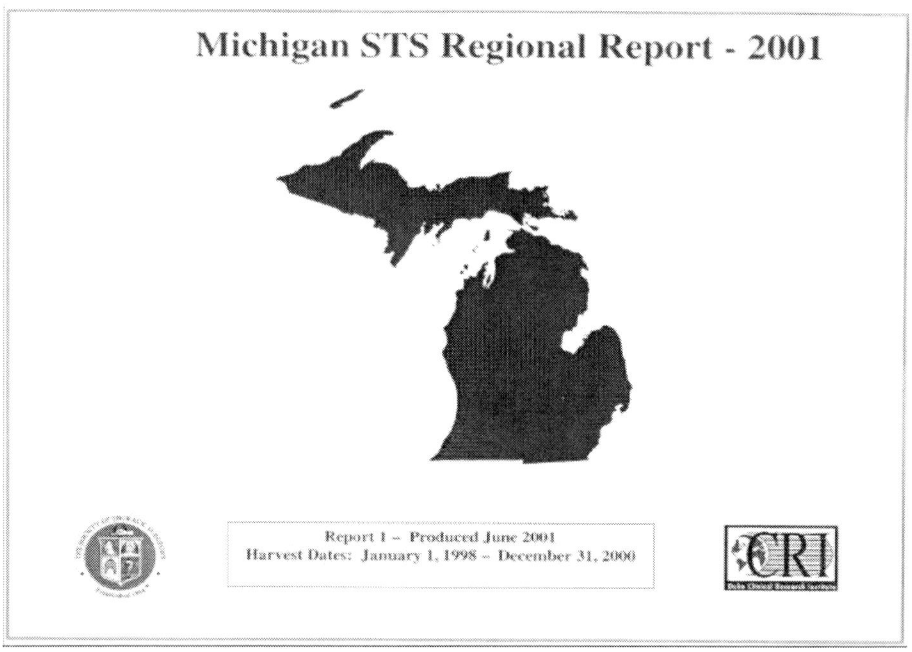
Michigan STS Regional Report - 2001
Report 1 – Produced June 2001
Harvest Dates: January 1, 1998 – December 31, 2000
CRI

Figure 6. This figure demonstrates the first page of the first STS report of comparative data for Michigan sites participating in the quality collaborative.

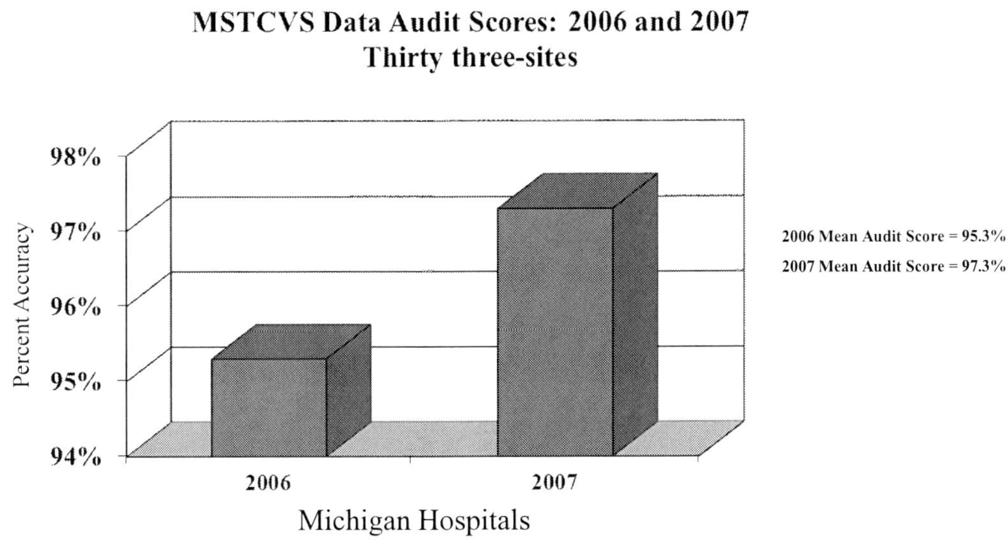

Figure 7. This figure shows the improvement in data quality with the initiation of site data audits.

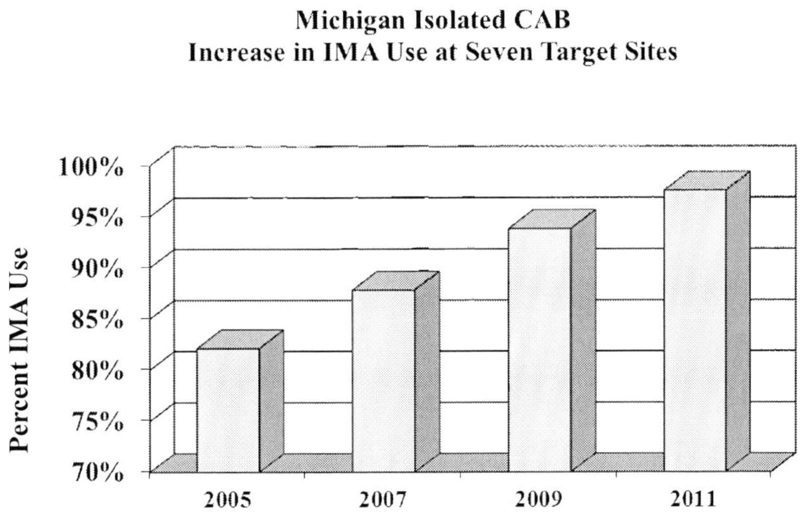

Figure 8. This figure demonstrates improvement of the 7 lowest sites of internal mammary artery utilization in Michigan from 2005 to 2011.

In Michigan as cardiac surgery sites became more comfortable reviewing and sharing data and outcomes, a fledgling quality collaborative arm of the MSTCVS began and requested comparative data for all participating programs. The first report was in 2001 with seventeen sites participating, Figure 6. The data were initially presented and discussed in blinded form at the summer meetings. By 2005 each Michigan cardiac surgery site voluntarily participated in the STS database and in our quality collaborative effort. Voluntary participation by all 33 sites in Michigan was a critical step in forming a statewide quality collaborative. Voluntary participation and a base of long term personal and professional relationships allowed for frank confidential discussions of site specific data on the meeting floor. Initially the data were presented in a blinded fashion so each site could see its data relative to the other sites. Over several years an atmosphere of non-critical and noncompetitive program improvement was fostered. Sites gradually became more comfortable allowing their data to be shared and discussed. Programs with exceptional results in one endpoint were asked to explain their process of care in this area. These practices were made available to all sites allowing allsites the opportunity to evaluate their own processes of care and adopt and implement new processes to strive for improvement. The review of these data and these discussions eventually became important additions to our annual meeting.

The MSTCVS entered discussions with Blue Cross/Blue Shield of Michigan to form a collaborative between a payer, physicians, and institutions. BCBS of Michigan is the dominant private insurer in Michigan. The discussions focused on maintaining the MSTCVS as owners of the collaborative data and the MSTCVS would lead the quality improvement initiative. BCBS would help fund the iniative and have access to blinded data and attendance at meetings. In 2005 with an agreement in place, BCBS of Michigan began to partially fund the cardiac-surgeon led quality collaborative.

The goals were:

1. Maintain a quality collaborative data system throughout the state for cardiac operations and maintain voluntary participation of all cardiac surgical programs
2. Creating mechanisms for review of appropriate data
3. Creating rapid cycle feedback for programs in the state using data
4. Funding full time personnel and a coordinating/resource center to create an audit system as well as an active communication system with all programs in the state
5. Funding for expenses at each institution for data management
6. Funding for quarterly reports and meetings

With funding, a central office was established and two nurses with STS data experience were hired, one designated as a data management specialist and one as a quality improvement specialist. Email communications across the state, a web site, and the arrangement of quarterly meetings were all established. A core group of experienced data managers from Michigan sites began to meet to improve statewide understanding of STS database definitions and coding of cases. [4] Quarterly meetings were rotated to participating program hospitals and attended by the surgeons and data managers. At each meeting state data was discussed and national experts presented regarding various aspects of quality or more directly on topics of care in cardiac surgery. Speakers from corporate America, NASA, and prominent cardiac surgeons have all participated at quarterly meetings. The coordinating center creates site visits to all programs to audit the quality of data input. Each site receives an audit score reflective of the accuracy of their data input. See Figure 7.

In Michigan, after creating our own state data warehouse utilizing one of the STS approved vendors, state data are analyzed with each harvest and available within two months to review at a quarterly meeting allowing evaluation of the quarterly performance of each site in selected outcome measures:

- Preoperative aspirin
- Preoperative Beta blocker
- Internal mammary artery use for conduit
- Postoperative prolonged ventilation
- Postoperative deep sterna wound infection
- Postoperative permanent CVA

- Postoperative renal failure
- Postoperative atrial fibrillation
- Postoperative reoperation for bleeding
- No red blood cell transfusion intra or postoperatively
- Beta blocker at discharge
- Anti-lipid medication at discharge
- 30 day readmissions
- Operative mortality

At quarterly meetings data on atheseendpoints as well as others arediscussed. All programs have two selected process improvement plans for chosen for each year. An early project was to increase use of the internal mammary artery (Lima) as conduit in isolated coronary bypass procedures. Use of the internal mammary confers reduced risk of mortality. [5] The seven sites of lowest utilizers of the internal mammary artery graft utilized a process-improvement plan to increase lima utilization. Lima use by the low utilizers increased from 82.0% to 92.7% from 2005 to 2008. See Figure 8. Use of the IMA in Michigan increased from 91.9% to 95.8% and is now higher than the STS database national average. [6] See Figure 9.

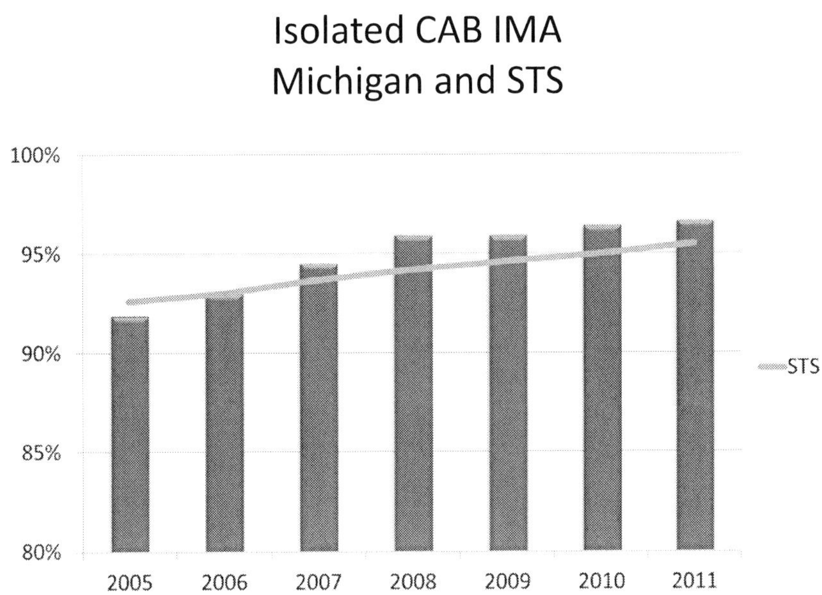

Figure 9. This figure demonstrates the improvement in utilization of internal mammary artery in CAB surgery in Michigan from 2005 to 2011.

Prolonged ventilation has been targeted as a quality improvement initiative. Prolonged ventilation (greater than 24 hours on ventilator after CAB) has been estimated to cost more than $30,000 dollars per event for hospitals. [7] See Figures 10 and 11. Other initiatives are directed at pre-operative intra-aortic balloon pump use, blood conservation (ref), post-operative atrial fibrillation, postoperative renal failure, postoperative stroke and readmission. Several sites have made dramatic progress in selected endpoints while participating in the collaborative. With regard to accomplishing correct discharge medication, the progress of the MSTCVS can be seen Figures 12 and 13.

Although the great majority of cardiac surgical procedures can be accomplished with a high degree of reliability and safety, the risk of mortality is ever present. The study of surgical mortalities is inherent in surgical training and remains paramount in our improvement efforts. In cardiac surgery death is often the end result of a cascade of decisions and events and clinicians from multiple disciplines may be involved in the care and decision making for an individual patientexperience.

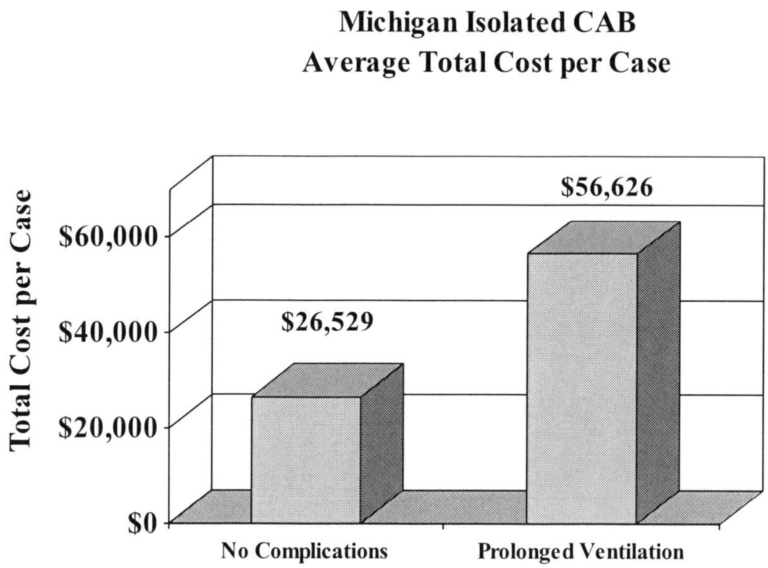

Figure 10. This figure demonstrates the financial impact of an episode of prolonged ventilation on cost of care for CAB patient.

Recognizing the efforts of the VA system in analyzing cardiac surgical mortalities as well as the Northern New England Cardiovascular study group) the MSTCVS, with the initiative and help of surgeons at one of our participating institutions, developed a phase of care mortality analyses (POCMA), a unique method for each program in Michigan to evaluate patient deaths. [8] This method has been adopted by all sites. For each death in Michigan the surgeon of record identifies the point in time where the inciting event for the mortality occurred. The events are grouped into one of five time frames. Phases of care such as preoperative, intraoperative, ICU, postoperative, and after discharge are all evaluated to determine when the inciting event preceding death occurred. In the preoperative phase issues such as patient risk factors, timing of surgery, patient preparations for surgery and patient risk versus benefit are evaluated. In the operating suite factors such as anesthesia management, surgeon decision making technical approaches, management of cardiopulmonary bypass are considered. After surgery, care in the ICU is evaluated by reviewing hemodynamic management, respiratory care, nutritional support, appropriate prophylaxis, glycemic control, recognition of decompensation, etc. On the step down unit issues such as anti-coagulation, rhythm management and nursing and physician observation and recognition of problems are all evaluated. After discharge patient medications, patient disposition, discharge destination, and patient support network are all considered. The intention of POCMA is to identify the root cause for the mortality and categorize the event in the appropriate phase of care and judge all events and deaths as avoidable or unavoidable.

Figure14 is an example of the Phase of Care Mortality Analysis (POCMA). Each institution forwards a POCMA form for each death to the MSTCVS Quality Collaborative coordinating center. The death is then reviewed by the Quality Committee. The committee has the option to accept the form as is or review the case in detail and change the final determinations. A phase of care mortality analysis summary is then returned to each institution profiling where most sentinel events occurred in their program. Local efforts can then be made to continue to eliminate avoidable deaths by improving processes of care and or making structural improvements where necessary.

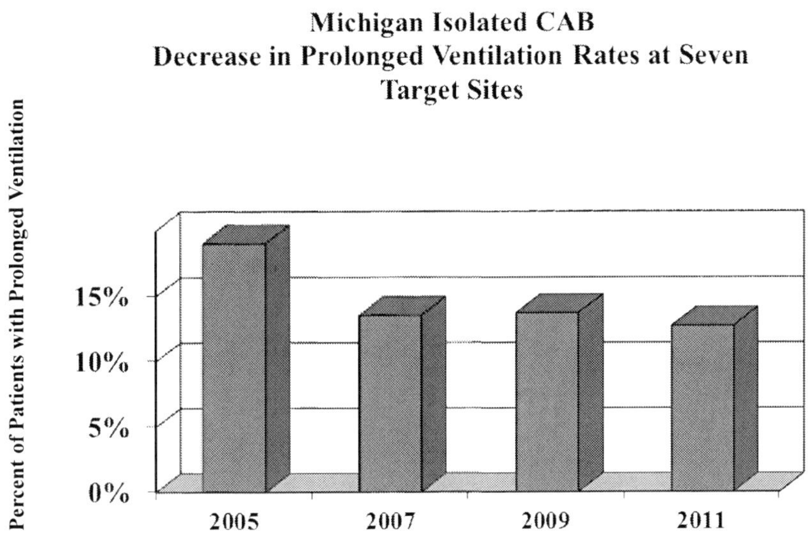

Figure 11. This figure shows the reduction in incidence of prolonged ventilation at the 7 worst performers in Michigan from 2005 to 2011.

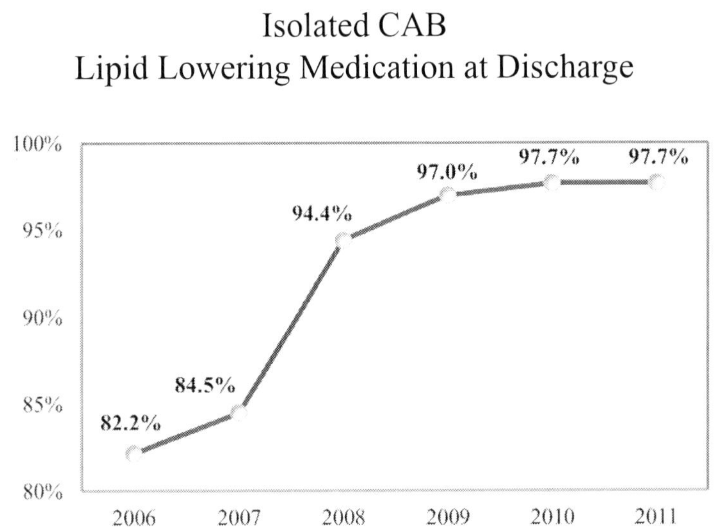

Figure 12. This figure demonstrates the improvement in utilization of lipid lowering medication at time of discharge.

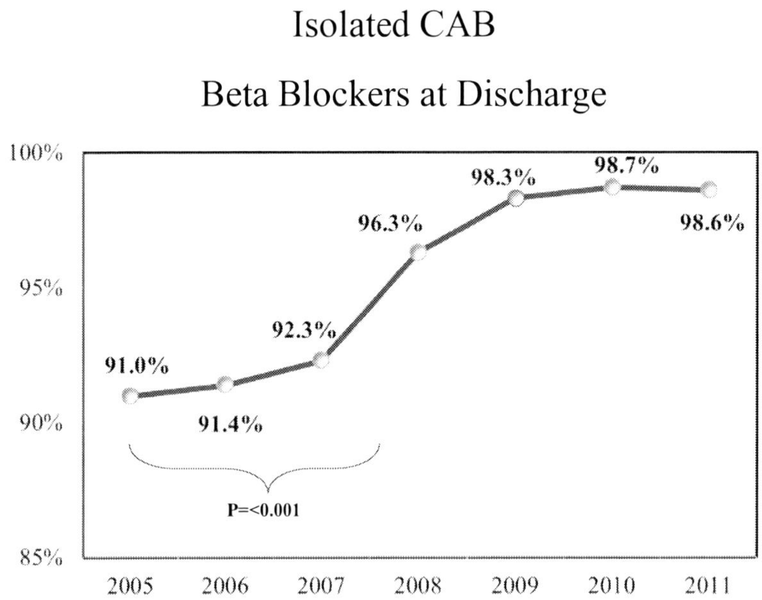

Figure 13. This figure demonstrates the improvement in utilization of Beta Blockers at time of discharge.

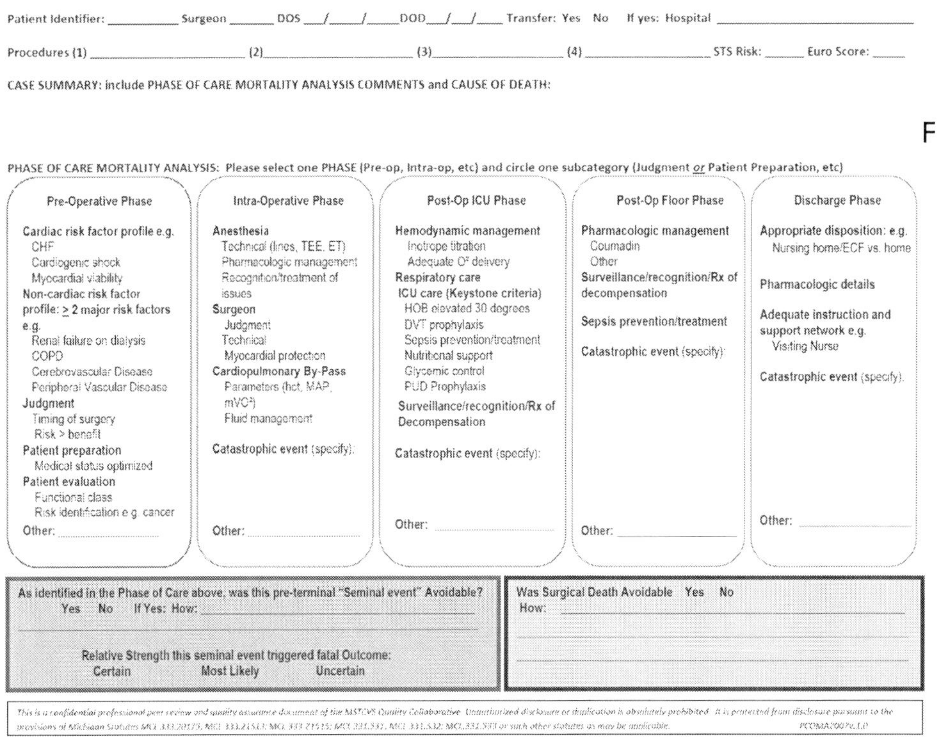

Patient Identifier: __________ Surgeon ______ DOS ___/___/___ DOD___/___/___ Transfer: Yes No If yes: Hospital ____________

Procedures (1) ______________ (2)______________ (3)______________ (4) ______________ STS Risk: ______ Euro Score: ______

CASE SUMMARY: include PHASE OF CARE MORTALITY ANALYSIS COMMENTS and CAUSE OF DEATH:

F

PHASE OF CARE MORTALITY ANALYSIS: Please select one PHASE (Pre-op, Intra-op, etc) and circle one subcategory (Judgment *or* Patient Preparation, etc)

Pre-Operative Phase

Cardiac risk factor profile e.g.
CHF
Cardiogenic shock
Myocardial viability
Non-cardiac risk factor profile: ≥ 2 major risk factors e.g.
Renal failure on dialysis
COPD
Cerebrovascular Disease
Peripheral Vascular Disease
Judgment
Timing of surgery
Risk > benefit
Patient preparation
Medical status optimized
Patient evaluation
Functional class
Risk identification e.g. cancer
Other: ______

Intra-Operative Phase

Anesthesia
Technical (lines, TEE, ET)
Pharmacologic management
Recognition/treatment of issues
Surgeon
Judgment
Technical
Myocardial protection
Cardiopulmonary By-Pass
Parameters (hct, MAP, mVO²)
Fluid management
Catastrophic event (specify):
Other: ______

Post-Op ICU Phase

Hemodynamic management
Inotrope titration
Adequate O² delivery
Respiratory care
ICU care (Keystone criteria)
HOB elevated 30 degrees
DVT prophylaxis
Sepsis prevention/treatment
Nutritional support
Glycemic control
PUD Prophylaxis
Surveillance/recognition/Rx of Decompensation
Catastrophic event (specify):
Other: ______

Post-Op Floor Phase

Pharmacologic management
Coumadin
Other
Surveillance/recognition/Rx of decompensation
Sepsis prevention/treatment
Catastrophic event (specify):
Other: ______

Discharge Phase

Appropriate disposition: e.g.
Nursing home/ECF vs. home
Pharmacologic details
Adequate instruction and support network e.g.
Visiting Nurse
Catastrophic event (specify):
Other: ______

As identified in the Phase of Care above, was this pre-terminal "Seminal event" Avoidable?
Yes No If Yes: How: ______________
Relative Strength this seminal event triggered fatal Outcome:
Certain Most Likely Uncertain

Was Surgical Death Avoidable Yes No
How: ______________

This is a confidential professional peer review and quality assurance document of the MSTCVS Quality Collaborative. Unauthorized disclosure or duplication is absolutely prohibited. It is protected from disclosure pursuant to the provisions of Michigan Statutes MCL 333.20175; MCL 333.21513; MCL 333.21515; MCL 331.531; MCL 331.532; MCL 331.533 or such other statutes as may be applicable.

Figure 14. This figure demonstrates a Phase Of Care Mortality Analysis (POCMA) form which is completed for each post cardiac surgery mortality in Michigan.

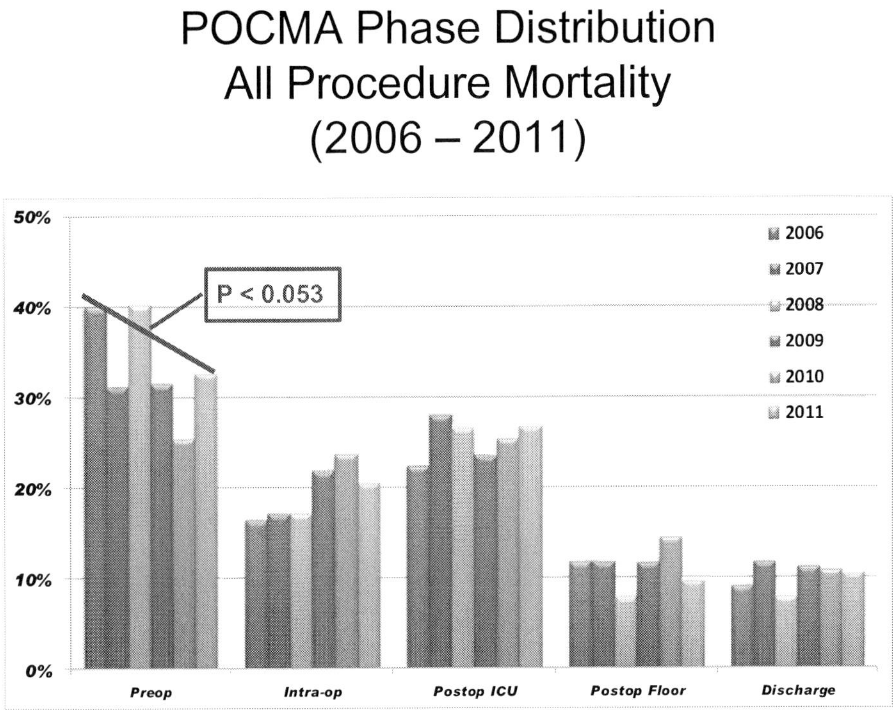

Figure 15. This figure demonstrates the distribution of mortality events by phase of care from 2006 to 2011.

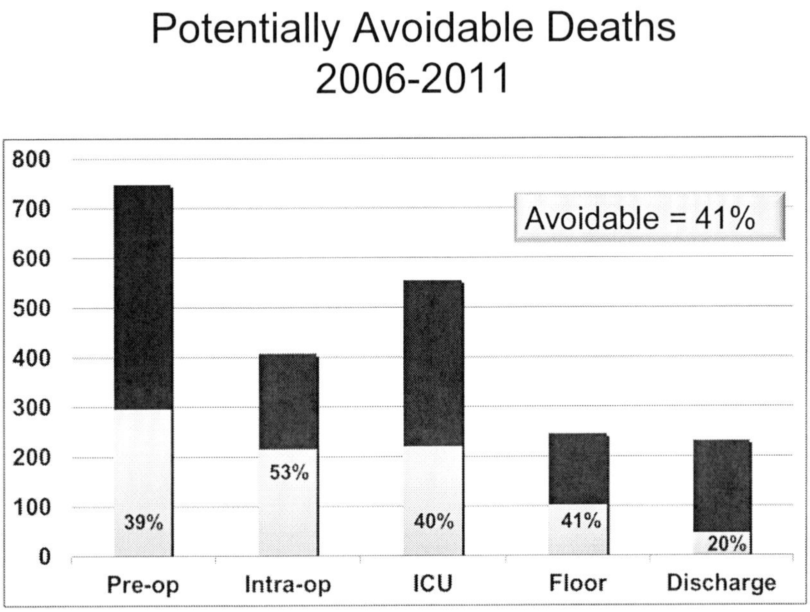

Figure 16. This figure demonstrates the proportion of post cardiac surgery deaths deemed avoidable after phase of care mortality analyses.

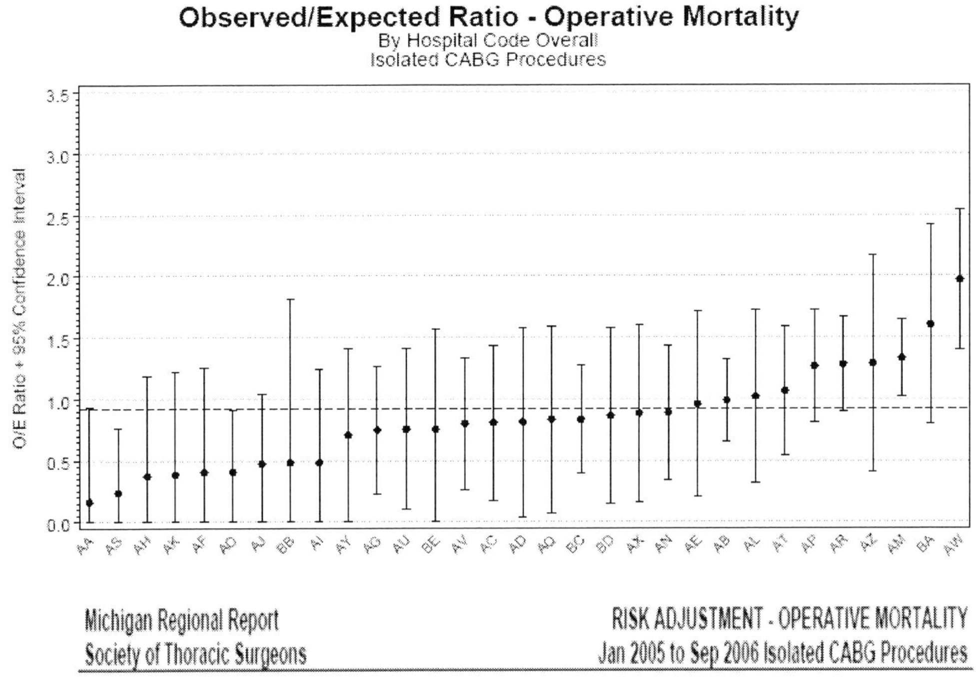

Figure 17. This figure demonstrates a typical mortality report showing the ratio of observed deaths at each institution versus the number of expected deaths based on their patient population. Originally the reports were blinded by site. Present reports are unblinded, but confidential to the discussants.

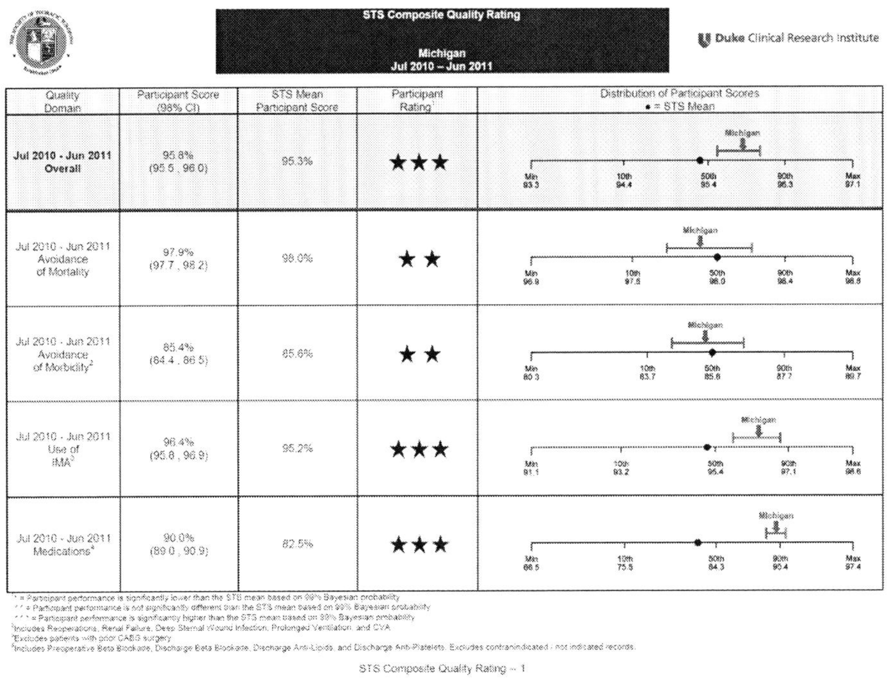

Figure 18. This figure demonstrates the 3-star composite rating for Michigan for 1 year ending June 2011.

POCMA was introduced in Michigan in 2006. Since 2007 POCMA has been conducted on all mortalities. Between January 1, 2006 and June 30, 2010, 53,674 adult cardiac operations were performed. Overall the most common phase of care where the death cascade was initiated was the preoperative phase (35%). 25% of inciting events were in ICU and 19% intra-operatively with 11% postoperatively and 10% after discharge. See Figure 15. In the preoperative phase the most common seminal events were patient cardiac risk factor profile, surgeon judgment regarding whether and when to operate, and patient noncardiac risk factor profile. Overall potentially avoidable mortality was 41% (729 of 1780). [9] See Figure16.

After individual mortality reviews are conducted locally and submitted, the regional report for Michigan showing the collective site-specific mortality results is presented at a quarterly meeting for discussion. When endpoints are graphically displayed for all sites, the range of performance can easily be seen. See Figure 17. Discussion may identify different processes of care or practice patterns which may be influencing outcomes. As seen by the above Figure, there are 10 sites with more observed than expected deaths. (We need to go over this and be certain the Committee is comfortable with this statement. Let's talk soon, RLP) These programs have opportunity to discuss their data and if the trend continues a site visit by surgeons from outside their referral area would occur. The collaborative coordinators plan, coordinate and participate in each site visit. The site visit is a process of preparation, interaction, education, and feedback. The process is described below:

PRE-VISIT REQUIREMENTS

Hospital

1. Complete patient mortality questionnaire (POCMA analysis, death summary, case data tool) for at least 10 cases. All deaths for previous calendar year (regardless of procedure type).
2. Assemble source documents for data that support POCM A analysis (e.g. ICU vital sign flow sheet for ICU event, cardiac catheterization for premature graft closure, PFTs for patient disease as primary cause of post-op respiratory failure).
3. Identify 2 areas for improvement on basis of POCMA trends for previous year.
4. Formulate quality improvement approach for these areas and summarize these recommendations for review by the reviewers.
5. Dream list: any and all changes in structural or process characteristics of the program that could result in improved survival for CAB only subset and CV surgery results in general.

Reviewers

1. Review death summaries, case data tool and POCMA
2. Comment on POCMA determinations (agree, disagree, questions for more data)
3. Identify 2 areas for improvement for program on basis of POCMA trends. Formulate suggestions for improvement.
4. Choose one unique case for presentation at state quality collaborative meeting that may provide a unique learning discussion.

SITE VISIT ATTENDANCE

Coordinating Center Quality and Data Nurses and Two Visiting Surgeons

Host Site Attendees

1. CV surgery chief and/or CV surgery quality "champion)" and institution surgeons
2. Lead cardiac anesthesiologist
3. Chief of cardiology
4. Chief of perfusion services
5. Head of ICU
6. Lead of physician extenders
7. Head nurses of ICU and step-down units
8. Data manager
9. Service line hospital administrator

GOAL: EVALUATE AND DESCRIBE THE PROGRAM WITHIN THE CONTEXT OF THE FOLLOWING VARIABLES

General information

- # cardiac catheterization and stents (PCI) and CAB surgery
- PCI vs. lytics for acute MI etc.

Operating Room

- Dedicated cardiac anesthesia?
- TEE certified?
- Anesthesiologist or CRNA?
- On-call OR staff dedicated heart team?
- Training of surgical assistants
- Hand-offs, Brief/Debrief

STANDARD PRE/POSTOP ORDERS

- Last update of standard orders
- Protocols for Atrial Fibrillation
- Other Protocols:

ICU

- Intensivist- board certified?
- Scope of in-house coverage:
- 24/7 (who covers evenings, nights)
- ICU Keystone Program?

Nursing

- Training of nursing staff.
- Nurse-patient ratio on days
- Nurse-patient ratio on afternoons & midnights
- Transfer to step-down, Hand-off

Physician Extenders

- PA's, NP's, RNFA's roles
- Chain of command, direction of surgeons

Performance Review

- M&M: process for review
- Monthly mortality conference
- Multidisciplinary
- Compliance with attendance

Cardiac Surgery Section Meetings

- Monthly conference
- Multidisciplinary
- Compliance with attendance
- Special Interests of CV surge

Dialogue

1. Discuss areas for improvement identified by reviewer and hospital. By discussion, drill down to 2 potential projects to improve outcomes in the coming year. Brainstorm to identify and list metric (s) to track and document progress or implementation of program.
2. Identify key structural variable (s) that should be modified to improve results and formulate letter to appropriate individual (s) to recommend change and rationale (e.g.

hospital administrator to fund 24/7 in house ICU coverage or chief of anesthesia to develop cardiac surgery specialization, etc.)
3. Establish relationships to foster continued communication between program and quality reviewers

VERIFICATION

1. Verify credentials and characteristics of program structural variables described on site questionnaire
2. Review protocols and standardized order forms

CONCLUSION

1. Re-state strengths and weaknesses of program in summary presentation by reviewers to all attendees
2. Summarize recommendations and comments of reviewers to group
3. Outline follow-up measures …… 6 and 12 month submission of POCMA results for subsequent mortalities and documented progress on quality improvement measures. Reverse Site visits are also available for surgeons and personnel from higher mortality programs to visit higher performing sites. By this approach sites are not left to struggle on their own to try to find remedies for their challenges but can benefit from input from the highest performers in the state. In addition to site visits we have utilized informative letters to sites who are underperforming in other endpoints such as high preoperative intra-aortic balloon pump use, stroke rate or prolonged ventilation.

As individual providers and as the MSTCVS Quality Collaborative, we are committed to delivering the safest, most efficient care we can. Reviewing our collaborative data revealed a fairly wide distribution of results, especially in the earlier years. Multiple strategies have been considered to reduce variation and improve quality of care. Public reporting of provider scorecards has been carefully scrutinized. The early practice of public reporting of unadjusted raw provider mortality was met with criticisms of overestimation of risk by providers, referring out high risk patients and withholding care from high risk patients. [10, 11, 12, 13, 14] To level the playing field, any publicly reported data should be by well-established national standards, audited for accuracy, and complemented by reporting measures of appropriateness. [15] The program composite data provided for the public by the STS is risk-adjusted, institution based, and reported voluntarily. The STS uses a three star system which should separate one, two, and three star performance with 99% probability that a true difference really exists.

A forum of voluntary collaboration can be effective way to raise the collective bar of performance. To have accurate risk stratification, there must be accurate reporting from all sites. If low performers choose not to report, the data pool is biased toward better outcomes. If all sites participate in a voluntary fashion learning, can occur across typical competitive barriers and a "learning community" created. The lessons learned from one site can be applied at a different site. Statewide collaboration allows similar sized programs or programs facing similar challenges to collaborate and share experiences rather than learn in isolation by trial and error.

In attempts to improve quality of care the structural components must be assessed as well as the process of care. Structural components such as size and type of institution (large, small, private, teaching hospital) as well rural or urban location may influence patient outcomes. In additions such factors as type of practice, amount of ancillary support, expertise of supporting services, utilization of computer orders and care plans may also be components which lend themselves to improved delivery of care. The Leapfrog group has identified computerized computer order entry, and presence of intensivists as markers for lower mortality (ref). The ultimate quality of the care delivered is derived from the interplay of the structural components of delivery and the conduct of the surgical procedure. Few structural components have been closely scrutinized as much as surgical volume. While some believe higher volume institutions with higher volume surgeons generally yield lower mortality [16, 17], there are unquestionably small programs withextremely low mortality as well. Alternatively high volume programs may exist with poor mortality scores. Quite possibly there are other recognized or unrecognized variables in the structure or delivery which are also important. While recognizing concrete outcomes such as mortality by surgeon or institution is an approach, the true challenge is in finding the factors that are important and putting the necessary structural components in an efficient process of care to deliver the best care to each patient undergoing a procedure.

The MSTCVS Quality Collaborative has accomplished a major milestone in elevating the collective performance of the entire state of Michigan to the upper echelon of national ranks.

During our earlier reporting periods (2006 and 2007) the collective performance of the Michigan sites when compared to the nation as a whole was not distinguishable. In our later reporting (2010-2011) Michigan as a whole achieved a 3 star rating from the Society of Thoracic Surgeons, demonstrating that within 99% probability we were performing approximately in the top decile of performance. See Figure 18.

Although most providers do not favor public reporting, we must realize that transparency of results is increasingly demanded by payers and patients and should be recognized by providers as a professional responsibility. As providers our quality collaborative members believe we are responsible within our specialty and institutions to raise the bar of performance to best serve our patients.

The unique situation of open discussion of site specific results among regional peers appears to be a strong motivator for change. Quarterly outcome discussions with all 33 peer groups provides for a great deal of regular input for results which can be very difficult to interpret in an isolated fashion. The MSTCVS Quality Collaborative has translated an interest in improving quality of care into demonstrated benefit for the patients in our state. While much work remains to be done there is much to be said for regional collaboration with focus on site specific goals to improve quality of care.

References

[1] Silbergleit A. A Brief History of the MSTCVS.
[2] http://www.sts.org/national-database.

[3] http://riskcalc.sts.org/STSWebRiskCalc273/About%20the%20STS%20Risk%20Calculator%20v2.73.pdf.

[4] Prager R. L., Armenti F. R., Bassett J. S., Bell G. F., Drake D., Hanson E. H., Heiser J. C., Johnson S. H., Plasmin F. B., Shannon F. L., Share D., Theurer P., Williams J. et al. Cardiac Surgeons and the Quality Movement: the Michigan Experience. *Thoracic and Cardiovascular Surgery* 2009;21:20-27.

[5] Loop F. D., Lytle B. W., Cosgrove D. M. et al. Influence of the Internal Mammary artery Graft on 10-year Survival and Other Cardiac Events. *N Engl J Med* 1986;314:1-6.

[6] Prager R. L., Armenti F. R., Bassett J. S. et al. Cardiac Surgeons and the Quality Movement: the Michigan Experience. *Semin Thorac Cardiovasc Surg* 21:20-27.

[7] Prager R. L., Armenti F. R., Bassett J. S. et al. Cardiac Surgeons and the Quality Movement: the Michigan Experience. *Semin Thorac Cardiovasc Surg* 21:20-27.

[8] Shannon F. L., Fazzalari F. L., Theure P. F., Bell G. F., Sutcliffe K. M., Prager R. L. A Method to Evaluate Cardiac Surgery Mortality: Phase of Care Mortality Analysis. *Annals of Thoracic Surgery* 2011 (in press).

[9] Shannon F. L., Fazzalari F. L., Theure P. F., Bell G. F., Sutcliffe K. M., Prager R. L. A Method to Evaluate Cardiac Surgery Mortality: Phase of Care Mortality Analysis. *Annals of Thoracic Surgery* 2011 (in press).

[10] Omoigui N. A., Miller D. P., Brown K. J., Annan K., Cosgrove D., Lytle B., Loop F., Topol E. Outmigration For Coronary Bypass in an Era of Public Dissemination of Clinical Outcomes. *Circulation* 1996;93 (1):27-33.

[11] Burack J. H., Impellizzeri P., Homel P., Cunningham J. N. Jr. Public Reporting of Surgical Mortality: A Survey of New York State Cardiothoacic Surgeons, *Annals of Thoracic Surgery*. 1999; 68:1195-1200.

[12] Narins C. R., Dozier A. M., Ling F. S. et al. The Influence of Public Reportin of Outcome Data on Medical Decision Makng by Physicians. *Arch Intern Med* 2005;165:83-87.

[13] Resnic F. S., Welt F. G. P. The Public Health Hazards of Risk Avoidance Associated With Public Reporting of Risk-Adjusted Outcomes in coronary Intervention. *JACC* 2009;53:825-30.

[14] Resnic F. S., Welt F. G. P. The Public Health Hazards of Risk Avoidance Associated With Public Reporting of Risk-Adjusted Outcomes in coronary Intervention. *JACC* 2009;53:825-30.

[15] Resnic F. S., Welt F. G. P. The Public Health Hazards of Risk Avoidance Associated With Public Reporting of Risk-Adjusted Outcomes in coronary Intervention. *JACC* 2009;53:825-30.

[16] Piet N. P., Kuijpers M., Zijlstra F. The relation between volume and outcome of coronary interventions: a systematic review and meta-analysis. *European Heart Journal* (2010) 31, 1985-1992.

[17] Hannan E. L., Wu C., Ryan T. J. et al. Do Hospitals and Surgeons With Higher Coronary Bypass Graft Surgery Volumes Still Have Lower Risk-Adjusted Mortality Rates? *Circ* 2003;108:795-801.

INDEX

C

D

E

F

G

H

I

J

K

L

M

Q

R

S

T

U

V

W

X

Y